T0289400

Cost-Benefit Analysis of Comprehensive Military Eye Examination Policies

RAFFAELE VARDAVAS, PHILIP ARMOUR, SAI PRATHYUSH KATRAGADDA,
TOYYA PUJOL-MITCHELL, PEDRO NASCIMENTO DE LIMA, BAQIR FATEH,
HELIN HERNANDEZ, STACEY YI, JAVIER ROJAS AGUILERA,
CATRIA GADWAH-MEADEN

Prepared for the Defense Health Agency Vision Center of Excellence
Approved for public release; distribution is unlimited.

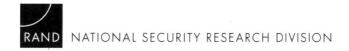

NATIONAL SECURITY RESEARCH DIVISION

For more information on this publication, visit **www.rand.org/t/RRA2188-1**.

About RAND

RAND is a research organization that develops solutions to public policy challenges to help make communities throughout the world safer and more secure, healthier and more prosperous. RAND is nonprofit, nonpartisan, and committed to the public interest. To learn more about RAND, visit www.rand.org.

Research Integrity

Our mission to help improve policy and decisionmaking through research and analysis is enabled through our core values of quality and objectivity and our unwavering commitment to the highest level of integrity and ethical behavior. To help ensure our research and analysis are rigorous, objective, and nonpartisan, we subject our research publications to a robust and exacting quality-assurance process; avoid both the appearance and reality of financial and other conflicts of interest through staff training, project screening, and a policy of mandatory disclosure; and pursue transparency in our research engagements through our commitment to the open publication of our research findings and recommendations, disclosure of the source of funding of published research, and policies to ensure intellectual independence. For more information, visit www.rand.org/about/research-integrity.

RAND's publications do not necessarily reflect the opinions of its research clients and sponsors.

About This Report

Vision readiness ensures that service members (SMs) have the visual fitness required to perform their missions successfully, maintain deployability, and serve without duty limitations. However, SMs may become ineligible for deployment due to ocular and visual dysfunctions (OVDs); and even if they are still eligible for deployment, their performance may suffer due to a lack of diagnosis or a lack of treatment for these dysfunctions. Moreover, if ocular/vision-related dysfunctions are not diagnosed and managed at an early stage, the cost of health care related to treating these dysfunctions increases.

While prior research has found that SMs are at high risk for OVDs, and particularly OVDs secondary to traumatic brain injuries (VDTBIs), current screening processes across all SMs focus on detecting and addressing refractive errors (REs) such as myopia, hyperopia, and astigmatism. As such, other OVDs that SMs are at risk for may go undiagnosed and untreated. In this report, we gather data and develop models to ascertain the costs and benefits of moving from the current visual acuity screening process for SMs to comprehensive eye examinations intended to detect a wider range of OVDs earlier, including dry eye, glaucoma, keratoconus, corneal dystrophies, retinal dystrophies, REs, and VDTBIs. Our model examines the costs and benefits of these comprehensive eye exams administered just after accession and periodically throughout service.

We draw on available data on the prevalence and incidence of these dysfunctions for the young adult U.S. population; factor in costs associated with exams, treatment, and discharges within the military context; and consider a range of values for the benefits of detecting otherwise undiagnosed OVDs among SMs. A central assumption of our model is that undiagnosed OVDs render SMs, on average, less productive, thereby diminishing the visual readiness value they add to the force. The primary benefit from comprehensive eye examinations is thus to detect and treat these dysfunctions, restoring full productivity. However, we find no widespread agreement on the expected impact of undiagnosed OVDs on productivity in the military. Because we would expect the impact of undiagnosed OVDs to vary by the nature of an SM's duties, from a minor inconvenience to the potential for active harm to the SM, unit, or mission, we do not assume a single value in our model. Instead, we provide cost-benefit analyses across a wide range of assumed negative impacts of undiagnosed OVDs. The intent of our research is not to show that any one of these assumed impacts on productivity is the "correct" impact but that the reader can observe how dependent the results are on this assumed negative impact and accordingly interpret the benefits of comprehensive eye exams for certain types of SMs.

Although our model is mathematically technical, the details of screenings and examinations for specific OVDs are medically technical, and the cost and benefit context requires knowledge of existing military policy, we have endeavored to write this report with a broader audience in mind, albeit one that has some familiarity with cost-benefit analyses and occupational limitations from visual disorders.

The research reported here was completed in March 2024 and underwent security review with the sponsor and the Defense Office of Prepublication and Security Review before public release.

RAND National Security Research Division

This research was sponsored by Defense Human Resources Activity, Office of the Under Secretary of Defense (OUSD) for Personnel and Readiness (P&R) and conducted within the Personnel, Readiness, and Health Program of the RAND National Security Research Division (NSRD), which operates the National Defense Research Institute (NDRI), a federally funded research and development center sponsored by the Office of the Secretary of Defense, the Joint Staff, the Unified Combatant Commands, the Navy, the Marine Corps, the defense agencies, and the defense intelligence enterprise.

For more information on the RAND Personnel, Readiness, and Health Program, see www.rand.org/nsrd/prh or contact the director (contact information is provided on the webpage).

Acknowledgments

We acknowledge the critical feedback from Sarah Meadows and Carter Price, our internal quality assurance reviewers for this project; and those from our external reviewer, Professor Sze-Chuan Suen of the University of Southern California. Daniel Ginsberg and Molly McIntosh's leadership at the NSRD provided invaluable comments, suggestions, and guidance. We furthermore emphasize the impossibility of undertaking this study without the feedback and subject matter expertise from the Vision Center of Excellence staff—most notably, our subject matter experts (SMEs), Rita Mallia and Michael Pattison; as well as David Eliason, CAPT Todd Lauby, COL Scott McClellan, and Patty Morris. We also thank SME support from the Tri-Service Vision Conservation & Readiness Program. Diane Egelhoff expertly prepared this document for review.

Summary

Ocular and visual dysfunctions (OVDs) encompass a range of conditions that can significantly affect an individual's vision and overall quality of life. OVDs can have significant implications for military personnel, particularly in terms of their readiness, performance, and overall well-being, and military personnel face disproportionately higher exposure to risk factors causing these dysfunctions, including traumatic brain injuries.

Currently, the only visual tests administered to all service members (SMs) are basic acuity screenings, which assess an SM's visual acuity (e.g., myopia, hyperopia, astigmatism) at entry and then periodically throughout service. However, these screenings do not capture the full range of OVDs that can affect military personnel, nor do they provide valuable baseline documentation on nonacuity visual conditions useful for diagnoses and treatment after subsequent service-related hazards. A comprehensive eye examination policy could provide significant benefits in diagnosing and treating dysfunctions sooner, establishing baseline measurements for future testing or the existence of preexisting conditions and optimizing warfighter readiness through occupational sorting.

However, administering comprehensive eye exams to all SMs would incur additional costs. In this study, we model whether the benefits of introducing baseline and periodic comprehensive eye exams for all SMs exceed their costs. We specifically focus on how comprehensive eye exams could increase detection of REs, as well as six other OVDs that current basic acuity screenings are not designed to detect: OVD secondary to traumatic brain injury, corneal dystrophies, retinal dystrophies, dry eye, keratoconus, and glaucoma. We model the benefits of comprehensive eye exams (early detection and successful treatment) relative to the costs of these exams, assuming that these exams were performed just after accession, as well as regularly every three, five, or eight years—frequencies selected based on the timing of cognitive screenings for different occupational specialties and for sensitivity analyses. We examine several kinds of costs, including the direct costs of comprehensive eye exams, treatment costs on positive diagnoses, discharge costs related to unsuccessful treatment, the resulting medical severance pay, and SM replacement costs. We note that this modeling effort was based on a range of assumptions, which we discuss throughout the report.

Our central finding is that, under a wide range of assumptions, **baseline and periodic comprehensive eye exams are cost-effective relative to current basic acuity screening**. That is, the average benefits for periodic comprehensive eye exams for all SMs exceed their costs given the inputs of our model. Furthermore, we find that more frequent exams are more cost-effective than less frequent exams, since these exams allow for earlier diagnoses of OVDs and more effective treatment. We therefore recommend periodic comprehensive eye examinations for all SMs, although the recommended frequency of these examinations may vary depending on the assumed impact of undiagnosed OVDs on force readiness.

A primary driver of our results is how we model the benefits of comprehensive eye exams. We do this by assuming that SMs contribute "visual readiness value" to the force while serving—that is, we assume a monetary value of an SM being fully visually fit in order to calculate a benefit from treating otherwise undiagnosed OVDs (thereby restoring the SM to full visual fitness). This use of the word *readiness* does not correspond to existing binary classifications of whether an SM is deployable or retainable, since we assume that absent these comprehensive eye exams, undiagnosed OVDs would continue to go undetected. We therefore use the term *visual readiness value* to correspond to what a fully visually fit SM would contribute to the total force, and hence calculate the expected loss if an SM has an undiagnosed and untreated OVD but continues to serve.

This expected loss will vary accordingly to the occupational specialty and responsibilities of each SM, and even within specialties with clear civilian equivalents, we found no consensus in our literature review or in consultation with subject matter experts (SMEs) on the productivity losses associated with undiagnosed OVDs. Therefore, we run our model across a wide range of scenarios of this value, including when OVDs only partially diminish readiness contributions of SM; where OVDs eliminate any contribution to force readiness; or where OVDs lead an SM to detract from total force readiness.[1] Across all these scenarios, we find that comprehensive eye exams are cost-effective, with benefits exceeding costs the most when an undiagnosed OVD not only reduces productivity but also causes active harm to the force, and when the value of an SM being fully visually fit is highest.[2]

We model benefits in terms of dollar values since costs of examinations are easily modeled via dollar values, corresponding to the TRICARE or purchased care costs of these comprehensive eye exams, treatment costs for each OVD, and replacement and discharge costs if treatment is unsuccessful. Our main findings focus on calculating the net monetary benefit (NMB) of these comprehensive eye examinations among a simulated group of 1,000 SMs, from their accession through up to 40 years of service—that is, relative to the current policy of basic acuity screenings, what is the additional monetary benefit accrued by comprehensive eye examinations minus the additional costs associated with these examinations for these 1,000 SMs throughout their service careers.

Figure S.1 depicts these ranges of results of the average NMB of comprehensive eye examinations relative to acuity screenings, assuming these comprehensive eye exams will be conducted just after accession and then at regular frequencies. We show results separately by scenarios assuming different exam frequencies (three, five, or eight years), full readiness value based on either enlisted or officer pay trajectories, and productivity loss scenarios (mild, moderate, or severe visual readiness impact). But even within each scenario, we face a range of plausible values for our other parameters, including incidence of OVDs among SMs, accuracy of comprehensive eye exams in diagnosing these OVDs, and treatment efficacy. As such, we run 300 simulations for each scenario with varying values of these inputs within their plausible ranges, producing a range of simulated net benefits and costs. The results

---

[1] We refer to these three scenarios as *mild visual readiness impact* (i.e., where undiagnosed SMs still contribute readiness value, but their contribution is reduced by half); *moderate visual readiness impact* (i.e., an undiagnosed OVD reduces the visual readiness value contributions of an SM completely to zero); and *severe visual readiness impact* (i.e., where undiagnosed SM *subtracts* from force readiness by one-half of their fully healthy visual readiness value).

[2] We quantify the value of full visual fitness with two scenarios: one using enlisted pay trajectories and the other using officer pay trajectories. We emphasize that these are not intended to be representative of all enlisted SMs and all officer SMs, respectively (e.g., an SM serving in the special forces may have a high value of full visual fitness, regardless of whether being enlisted or being an officer—i.e., an enlisted drone pilot may have a high value of full visual fitness, whereas a judge advocate general officer may have a lower value). Instead, they are meant to be illustrative of how variation in the assumed full visual fitness level affects our findings.

depicted in Figure S.1 therefore summarize the range of net monetary value (net benefits minus net costs) from these simulations via both "box plots" (the median value and interquartile range [twenty-fifth to seventy-fifth percentiles of our simulated results]), as well as "violin plots," or the distribution of results, specifically the empirical probability distribution function. When these "violins" appear wider corresponds to a greater fraction of our simulations that corresponded to that value.

As shown in Figure S.1, there is a positive net monetary value of moving to a comprehensive eye exam policy relative to current screening policy across the different scenarios examined; the benefits nearly always exceed the costs. Comprehensive eye exams are most cost-effective when the assumed impact of an undiagnosed OVD on readiness is most severe. More frequent—every three years—eye exams tend to be slightly more cost-effective than less frequent exams; the similarity between results from different exam frequencies arises from more frequent exams diagnosing and treating OVDs sooner, yielding greater benefits, but also requiring substantially more exams with correspondingly greater exam costs. For the scenario based on enlisted pay, dividing the NMB for three-year exams by the 1,000 SM simulated population yields a median NMB of just over $200 per SM, given the most severe impact of OVDs on readiness; approximately $125 per SM, given the middle assumption over the impact of OVDs on readiness; and approximately $75 per SM, given the least assumed impact of OVDs on readiness. These net benefits are even higher in the scenario based on officer pay.

Based on our analysis, we recommend that SMs across all services undergo periodic comprehensive eye exams. We note that there is a range of plausible values of our modeling inputs due to a lack of representative and comparable estimates of prevalence, incidence, treatment effectiveness, testing specificity, testing sensitivity, and impacts on visual readiness value from published academic literature. However, across a broad array of assumptions, periodic comprehensive eye exams are cost-effective relative to current acuity screening policy, especially for SMs with high value of full visual fitness and the large expected negative impacts of undiagnosed OVDs on productivity. We note finally that we did not include the full range of potential benefits of comprehensive eye exams at accession and throughout service due to difficulty in quantifying them—namely, improved accuracy in establishing service connectedness of OVDs during the Veterans Affairs disability claims process, improved OVD diagnostic accuracy throughout an SM's career due to improved baseline measures, reduced medical spending due to early detection and successful treatment, and improved sorting into occupational specialty through this comprehensive baseline examination. Adding these benefits would increase the cost-effectiveness of comprehensive eye exams even more than our model suggests, further justifying our recommendation to introduce baseline and periodic comprehensive eye exams for all SMs.

Figure S.1. Net Monetary Cost per 1,000 Enlisted Service Members of Different Comprehensive Eye Exam Policies Relative to Current Acuity Screening Policy, by Assumed Impact of Undiagnosed Ocular and Visual Dysfunction on Visual Readiness and by Full Readiness Value

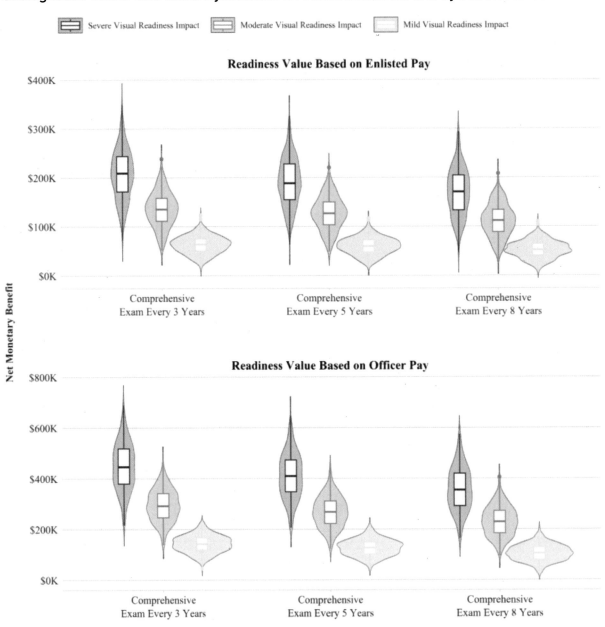

NOTE: Color coding corresponds to the assumed impact of an undiagnosed OVD on visual readiness values. Green corresponds to *mild visual readiness impact* (i.e., where undiagnosed SMs still contribute readiness value but their contribution is reduced by half); blue to *moderate visual readiness impact* (i.e., an undiagnosed OVD reduces the visual readiness value contributions of an SM completely to zero); and red to *severe visual readiness impact* (i.e., where undiagnosed OVD subtracts from force readiness by one-half of an SM's fully healthy visual readiness value).The y-axis is the NMB, our measure of cost-effectiveness, resulting from undertaking exam policy under consideration across the 1,000 SMs and 300 simulated runs, and hence shows total dollar figures for every 1,000 SMs. Box plots indicate the interquartile range (white rectangle) and median (a horizontal line in this rectangle), while violin plots show probability density function based on all runs of each policy frequency and readiness value reduction scenario. We vary the value of full visual readiness illustratively based on either average enlisted or officer pay trajectories.

Contents

Figures and Tables

Figures

Tables

Chapter 1

Introduction and Background

Ocular and visual dysfunction (OVD) encompasses a range of conditions that significantly affect individuals' vision, with direct consequences for productivity and quality of life. Among the most common forms of OVD are REs such as myopia, hyperopia, and astigmatism that directly affect individuals' visual acuity. However, there is a range of other conditions that can impair vision, and though these conditions are, in general, less common than REs, if undiagnosed and thus untreated, they can have both short- and long-term consequences for individuals' visual health.

The motivation for this study is that although service members (SMs) undergo regular basic acuity screenings intended to detect REs, not all SMs receive comprehensive eye examinations that would detect other OVDs. Yet SMs are exposed to a range of hazards that increase the risk of OVDs, including traumatic brain injuries (TBIs), as well as direct ocular damage. Given the lack of periodic comprehensive eye exams, some OVDs are thus likely to go undiagnosed and untreated, despite timely treatment improving visual fitness. We therefore model the costs and benefits of adding comprehensive eye exams to current basic acuity screening policies.

In this chapter we discuss the difference between comprehensive eye exams and basic acuity screenings, current military visual screening and exam policies, recent evidence-based recommendations for regular comprehensive eye exams based on the occupational burden of undiagnosed OVDs, and, finally, our analytic approach to modeling a change to military eye exam policy.

Comprehensive Eye Examinations and Current Policy

When we refer to *comprehensive eye examinations*, we use the guidelines of the American Optometric Association (AOA):

> A comprehensive adult eye and vision examination should include, but is not limited to:
>
> - Patient and family history, including visual, ocular, and general health, medication usage, and vocational and avocational visual requirements
> - Measurement of visual acuity
> - Determination of refractive status
> - Assessment of ocular motility, binocular vision, and accommodation, as appropriate, based on patient's age, visual signs, and symptoms
> - Ocular health examination, including evaluation of the anterior and posterior segments, measurement of intraocular pressure, and visual field testing

- Systemic health assessment, as indicated
- Ancillary testing, as needed.[3]

Current military policy includes measurement of visual acuity at accession and as part of SMs' annual Periodic Health Assessments.[4] This measurement is performed via a vision screening, whereby the SM reads an eye chart from a specified distance; in the event of a failure, there is a further determination of refractive status. Thus, although basic acuity screenings under current policy include "measurement of visual acuity" and subsequent "determination of refractive status," they do not include the other elements listed in the comprehensive eye exam description above. Given the acuity-focused medical requirements for accession, retention, and deployment,[5] these vision screenings are intended to detect refractive errors (REs).

Comprehensive eye exams are designed to diagnose a wide range of OVDs, and the AOA guidelines recommend *annual* comprehensive eye exams for all adults, including those ages 18 to 39. The guidelines note that "the educational, vocation and avocational visual requirements for individuals in this age group are substantial" and that although

> the prevalence of ocular disease is relatively low for young adults . . . many eye diseases can initially develop without signs or symptoms . . . to ensure early detection of potentially sight-threatening vision disorders, and for young adults to maintain their visual efficiency and productivity, periodic examinations are needed.[6]

There has long been recognition that the current vision screening policies of the U.S. Department of Defense (DoD) do not detect a substantial number of SMs with OVDs that may render them not visually ready, and that nearly half of SMs have *never* received a comprehensive eye exam.[7] Currently, SMs receive comprehensive eye exams if they present to a physician with damage to the eye or another

---

[3] AOA, *Comprehensive Adult Eye and Vision Examination: Evidence-Based Clinical Practice Guidelines*, 2nd ed., 2022, p. 12.

[4] Health.mil, "Periodic Health Assessment," undated.

[5] Per Department of Defense Instruction 6130.03, Volume 1, Section 6.4 ("Vision"), the following are vision-related disqualifying conditions for accession of an SM:

> a. Current distant visual acuity of any degree that does not correct with spectacle lenses to at least 20/40 in each eye.
> b. For entrance into Service academies and officer programs, the individual DoD Components may set additional requirements. The DoD Components will determine special administrative criteria for assignment to certain specialties.
> c. Current near visual acuity of any degree that does not correct with spectacle lenses to at least 20/40 in the better eye.
> d. Current refractive error (hyperopia, myopia, astigmatism) in excess of -8.00 or +8.00 diopters spherical equivalent or astigmatism in excess of 3.00 diopters.
> e. Any condition that specifically requires contact lenses for adequate correction of vision, such as corneal scars and opacities and irregular astigmatism.
> f. Color vision requirements will be set by the individual DoD Components.

DoD, *Medical Standards for Military Service: Appointment, Enlistment, or Induction*, Department of Defense Instruction 6130.03, Vol. 1, November 16, 2022. See also DoD, Office of the Actuary, *Valuation of the Medicare-Eligible Retiree Health Care Fund*, January 2022.

[6] AOA, 2022, p. 36.

[7] R. S. Buckingham, L. L. Cornforth, K. J. Whitwell, and R. B. Lee, "Visual Acuity, Optical, and Eye Health Readiness in the Military," *Military Medicine*, Vol. 168, No. 3, March 2003; R. S. Buckingham, D. McDuffie, K. Whitwell, and R. B. Lee, "Follow-Up Study on Vision Health Readiness in the Military," *Military Medicine*, Vol. 168, No. 10, October 2003.

ocular condition, request or are referred for an exam based on visual difficulties, or have persistence of an OVD after a TBI for at least two weeks. Although these exams are available through TRICARE or authorized purchased care, there is a selection effect of who seeks out or is referred to these exams. Relying on historical military health records to estimate prevalence and incidence of OVDs will thus result in an undercounting of OVDs among SMs. Furthermore, estimates of prevalence and incidence of OVDs based on nonmilitary populations are likely to be uninformative for the SM population. On the one hand, SMs tend to be physically healthier on average than civilian young adults, since they must satisfy physical and medical accession standards, and thus we may expect lower prevalence at accession. However, evidence from the academic literature on the incidence of OVDs indicates that risks vary widely by occupational setting and geography.[8] SMs have higher rates of exposure to physical risks and austere environments than civilians, which may thus substantially increase the incidence of OVDs.

The introduction of periodic comprehensive eye exams would therefore allow for accurate and representative diagnoses of OVDs. In this study, we identify six additional OVDs that, in interviews with military vision policy subject matter experts (SMEs), represent the greatest risk of undiagnosed occupational burden or for which early detection is particular important: corneal dystrophies, retinal dystrophies, dry eye, glaucoma, keratoconus, and OVD secondary to a TBI (VDTBI), including convergence insufficiency, accommodative dysfunction, and loss of visual field.

The Burden of Ocular and Visual Dysfunction

In this section, we focus on the consequences of OVDs for SMs' visual readiness. The AOA recommendations cited above for annual comprehensive eye exams for all adults ages 18 to 39 are evidence based. However, that evidence base draws from studies of occupational burden of OVD for all adults in the United States, and not specifically the SM population, which, as discussed above, may differ substantially in terms of prevalence and incidence of OVDs from the general population, as well as for the impact of OVDs on occupational performance.

However, there is a small amount of literature focused on the high incidence of TBIs among SMs in the last several decades that estimates the occupational burden of VDTBIs among SMs;[9] we thus consulted this literature to explore the potential burden of our wider set of OVDs for SMs. However, we found that these studies made assumptions over productivity losses associated with low vision based on civilian or older adult populations using dated empirical methodologies. For example, the 2019 study by Frick and Singman relies on Rein and colleagues' point-in-time differences in employment and earnings between adults ages 40–64 reporting low vision or blindness compared

---

[8] D. B. Rein, J. S. Wittenborn, P. Zhang, F. Sublett, P. A. Lamuda, E. A. Lundeen, and J. Saaddine, "The Economic Burden of Vision Loss and Blindness in the United States," *Ophthalmology,* Vol. 129, No. 4, April 2022; S. S. Islam, E. J. Doyle, A. Velilla, C. J. Martin, and A. M. Ducatman, "Epidemiology of Compensable Work-Related Ocular Injuries and Illnesses: Incidence and Risk Factors," *Journal of Occupational and Environmental Medicine,* Vol. 42, No. 6, June 2000.

[9] R. S. Buckingham, K. J. Whitwell, and R. B. Lee, "Cost Analysis of Military Eye Injuries in Fiscal Years 1988–1998," *Military Medicine,* Vol. 170, No. 3, March 2005; N. Merezhinskaya, R. K. Mallia, D. Park, D. W. Bryden, K. Mathur, and F. M. Barker II, "Visual Deficits and Dysfunctions Associated with Traumatic Brain Injury: A Systematic Review and Meta-Analysis," *Optometry and Vision Science,* Vol. 96, No. 8, August 2019; K. D. Frick and E. L. Singman, "Cost of Military Eye Injury and Vision Impairment Related to Traumatic Brain Injury: 2001–2017," *Military Medicine,* Vol. 184, Nos. 5–6, 2019.

with respondents who reported no difficulty seeing.[10] Although we conducted our own analysis of the productivity effects of low vision, as reported in Appendix C, we found that there was considerable variation in the literature and among SMEs consulted as to what the average burden may be, as well as how the burden is likely to vary by occupational specialty and age. Given this variability among SMs and lack of expert consensus, we therefore conduct analyses across a wide range of assumptions as to the burden of undiagnosed OVDs on SMs visual readiness. We now turn to discussing the details and assumptions of our microsimulation model.

Our Analytic Approach

A key objective of the project was to quantify the cost-effectiveness of eye exam policies to optimize vision readiness and ocular/vision care provided to SMs. We developed a microsimulation model—that is, a model that simulates each SM in a population individually, allowing us to conduct cost-benefit and cost-effectiveness analyses across a range of policy scenarios and assumptions. Our key research question is: Do the benefits of improved readiness from diagnosis and treatment of OVDs outweigh the costs of conducting comprehensive eye exams relative to the current basic acuity screening policy? Specifically, we model the introduction of a comprehensive eye exam administered to all SMs just after accession, as well as periodically at three-, five-, or eight-year intervals (maintaining annual vision screenings as part of Periodic Health Assessments). These intervals were chosen to align with existing cognitive screening policies for special forces SMs (three years) and other SMs (five years), with the eight-year frequency chosen to provide additional insight on the role of frequency of exams in determining their cost-effectiveness.

Essential to the strength of any modeling exercise is the realism of the inputs into the model. We informed these inputs through literature reviews and discussions with SMEs. We discuss the model inputs at length in Chapter 2, but we note here that because of the topic of our study—an examination of the costs and benefits of comprehensive eye exams relative to current acuity screening policy—there are simply not representative data on incidence and prevalence of OVDs among SMs. And, as is discussed in Chapter 4, there is considerable expected variation in the burden of undiagnosed OVDs among SMs.

When parameter values are known, we include specific values (e.g., medical discharge costs based on pay and years of service (YOS), and treatment costs through TRICARE). When these values are based on estimates from the civilian medical, social science, or military medicine research literatures (e.g., the prevalence of OVDs among young adults, or the incidence of TBIs among SMs), we allow our inputs to vary within a range based on the strength and applicability of this evidence, as discussed in Chapter 2 and documented in Appendix D. When values are unavailable, we use even larger ranges or set up separate scenarios to demonstrate how reliant our findings are on these alternatives. We accordingly provide caveats to our findings and recommendations, but we note again that our central finding—that the expected benefits of comprehensive eye exams for all SMs outweigh the expected costs—holds across nearly all scenarios and sensitivity analyses. We also note that any introduction of

---

[10] Frick and Singman, 2019; D. B. Rein, P. Zhang, K. E. Wirth, P. P. Lee, T. J. Hoerger, N. McCall, R. Klein, J. M. Tielsch, S. Vijan, and J. Saaddine, "The Economic Burden of Major Adult Visual Disorders in the United States," *Archives of Ophthalmology*, Vol. 124, No. 12, December 2006.

systematic comprehensive eye exam policy, even on a small but representative subset of SMs, would immediately provide valuable information to aid in modeling broader changes to eye exam policies across services.

The Organization of This Report

Chapter 2 describes the structure and operation of our microsimulation model and the formulation of the parameter inputs of the model, including the literature reviews we undertook and discussions with SMEs. Chapter 3 discusses the output of our modeling runs and the cost-benefit and cost-effectiveness results of different eye examination policies. Chapter 4 concludes by summarizing our findings, providing recommendations, and noting the major assumptions and caveats of our analytic approach. We provide the exact numerical results underlying the figures shown in the report in Appendix A and report the results of sensitivity analyses in Appendix B. Appendix C provides an alternative approach to estimating productivity loss from the onset of low vision compared with estimates in the literature that have limited applicability to our policy context. Finally, Appendix D documents all of our modeling inputs, their assumed ranges, and the sources we used to determine these values or ranges.

Chapter 2

Modeling the Dynamics of Visual Disorders Under Different Eye Examination Policies

Introduction

This chapter introduces a novel model that simulates the dynamics of independent OVDs within a population cohort of SMs and discusses its modeling inputs. Our model is a discrete-time microsimulation model that follows SMs at the individual level as they age, advancing with a yearly time step. The model tracks the visual readiness value that an SM contributes to the force in each year of service; an undiagnosed OVD detracts from this visual readiness value. Our model is designed to simulate the same cohort of SMs under different OVD examination policies, allowing decisionmakers to compare readiness outcomes with policy costs via a cost-benefit analysis (CBA), including basic acuity screening and various comprehensive eye exam policies. We simulate SMs who differ by their *full visual readiness value*, which assigns a monetary value to an SM's optimal visual health and which we quantify as following the average pay trajectory by YOS for either an enlisted or officer SM. We conduct further sensitivity analyses in which we assume higher multiples of these values. Additionally, we vary our assumed impact of an undiagnosed OVD on visual readiness value, from *mild* (reducing the annual visual readiness value contribution by one-half), to *moderate* (reducing it to zero), to *severe* (whereby the undiagnosed OVD subtracts from the force one-half of their full visual readiness value). The chief benefit from administering a comprehensive eye exam is to diagnose and treat an OVD that would otherwise go undiagnosed, thereby restoring the SM's full visual readiness value contribution to the force.

However, our model assumes that there may be errors in diagnoses, with lower test *specificity* resulting in more false positives (i.e., incorrect diagnosis in the absence of an OVD) and lower test *sensitivity* resulting in a higher probability of false negatives (i.e., failure to diagnose an OVD when it is present). The model then simulates the dynamics of OVDs and the incidence of TBI for each recruited SM as they progress through their service. We allow for SM attrition according to average attrition rates, with the vast majority of SMs leaving service before the age of 40.

An SM diagnosed with a condition is treated for their OVD. Treatment efficacy depends on the age at diagnosis and, if effective, is assumed to be permanently effective until the age that the SM separates. If the treatment is ineffective, we assume that the SM is discharged and replaced by the next most senior SM, who in turn is replaced by the next most senior SM, and so on. Ultimately, an additional SM needs to be recruited to maintain end strength. As such, we model the costs of ineffective treatment as not only the costs associated with discharging the SM with the OVD but also the additional replacement and training costs associated with recruiting and training a new SM. We model the costs of exams and treatment as well. The OVDs we consider are shown in Table 2.1.

Table 2.1. Modeled Ocular and Visual Dysfunctions and Risk Factors

Condition	Risk Factor
VDTBI	Individual TBI
Corneal dystrophy	Population average
Retinal dystrophy	Population average
RE	Population average
Dry eye	Population average
Keratoconus	Population average
Glaucoma	Population average

SOURCES: K. J. Ishak, N. Kreif, A. Benedict, and N. Muszbek, "Overview of Parametric Survival Analysis for Health-Economic Applications," *PharmacoEconomics*, Vol. 31, No. 8, August 2013; S. J. Richards, "A Handbook of Parametric Survival Models for Actuarial Use," *Scandinavian Actuarial Journal*, Vol. 2012, No. 4, 2012.

In our model, the probability that an SM is stricken with one of these seven OVDs is based on the population average, although for VDTBI, there is an additional risk factor (RF) to consider: having had at least one TBI. A TBI can, in some cases, lead to a VDTBI, including convergence insufficiency, accommodative dysfunction, or loss of field of vision. Our model thereby simulates not just the incidence of the above conditions based on our review of the scientific literature but also the incidence of TBI in order to inform the incidence of VDTBI. An observed TBI therefore immediately leads to a comprehensive eye exam in our model. Hence, our model includes policies through which SMs with a history of TBIs are screened more frequently. Additionally, we model the incidence of TBI *during service* as an RF that affects incidence of OVD. Unlike VDTBI, which is associated with a specific RF, the other six OVDs do not have an associated RF in our model.

Our model can separately consider different groups of SMs in separate runs, and parameter values specifying the model settings can be adjusted to reflect various types of SM, although the results in this report correspond to model runs based on a common range of parameters. Moreover, the seven OVDs we model are assumed to be independent, which means that an SM who has one or more conditions is equally as likely to develop an additional OVD as an SM with none of the OVDs listed in the table. This assumption has significant consequences, particularly in terms of comprehensive eye exams for all seven conditions. Since the OVDs are independent, it leads to increased false positive rates during the examination process. While the conditions are modeled as independent in our analysis, we acknowledge that there may be associations or comorbidities between some of the OVDs in real-world clinical scenarios. If literature or data can be found showing how frequently these conditions are diagnosed together among SMs, they could provide valuable context for understanding the potential for false positives in our modeling approach. Indeed, any systematic comprehensive eye exam policy implemented by DoD would provide valuable information on not just the prevalence of each OVD but also the comorbidity of OVDs among SMs. This information could help refine our interpretation of the results and improve the accuracy of our model predictions.

Simplifying Assumptions

In this section, we describe the assumptions underlying our model. Many of these parameters have a wide range of values, as described in the literature. Our simulation model should thus be viewed not as a tool for forecasting but rather to compare policies relative to each other and find which policies consistently outperform others under different assumptions. By exploring a multitude of model outcomes using unique combinations of plausible parameter values simulated within (otherwise known as *sampling from*) their estimated plausible ranges, we can identify which policies consistently outperform others while being robust to the underlying uncertainties.

Our model considers varying OVD incidence by age and determines the risks associated with developing OVDs, as well as the RF associated with VDTBI, the treatment efficacy for an OVD, and—because with age comes more YOS—the readiness value of an SM. We run our model over a range of assumptions of full visual readiness value (linked to enlisted or officer pay trajectories) and the severity of undiagnosed OVDs in order to show how dependent our findings are on the reader's assumed importance of the impact of undiagnosed OVDs on the force.

The impact of YOS on incidence is of key importance to our model, and we directly model how YOS affect incidence of OVDs. Additionally, as SMs age, they may separate from service because an OVD that is no longer treatable or through an age-dependent all-other-cause attrition rate. This latter rate accounts for background attrition effects that are unrelated to the SMs' vision fitness, including separating at the end of the term of service, retirements, disciplinary discharges, or other (non-vision-related) medical discharges.

The initial population cohort consists of a number (N) of SMs entering the military at age 18; we note that we use age values for primarily illustrative, not substantive, purposes. Years of service are substantially more important in our model, since changes in visual readiness values and incidence of OVDs and TBIs are related directly to YOS. Our model results would be largely unchanged if we simulated SMs starting at any point from ages 17 to 29.

Typically, we set N to 1,000, since this size allows for sufficient incidence of OVDs, is not so large as to make model runs intractable, and makes aggregate numbers easily interpretable. Therefore, our model's prediction intervals encompass a range of outcomes expected in each simulation of 1,000 SMs. The model independently simulates the same population over a large range of unique combinations of input parameter values and policy settings, specifying the number of case runs (M) of our experimental design, which in our analyses is set to 300. To explore the effects of different input parameter values and screening versus examination policies, we need to simulate a large range of unique combinations in our experimental design. Therefore, the number of independent cases M is set high at 300 to account for variabilities resulting from changes in model parameter values rather than stochastic, chance-driven variabilities seen in individual case runs. Simulating too few SMs in a single run would lead to excessive stochastic variability, while excessively large values of N would result in longer simulation times, limiting the size of M and the overall exploration range and density. The model is also specified by the maximum age that an SM can serve, which we set to 60. However, given our all-other-cause attrition rates, most SMs separate by age 40, and the majority of our age-based parameter inputs stay fixed after age 40.

Policy Assumptions and Inputs

The current testing practice for SMs is a basic acuity screening conducted at baseline and periodically at annual intervals. This screening is primarily used for detecting REs. In our model we assume that the accuracy of detecting REs is lower for the basic acuity screening compared with the comprehensive eye exam. That is, the specificity value for the basic acuity screening is lower than that for the comprehensive eye exam. This means that the basic acuity screening is more likely to incorrectly identify SMs as having REs (false positives) compared with the comprehensive eye exam. We model the costs and benefits of this current screening policy.

We then model our alternative policies that add to this existing screening policy—namely, administering *comprehensive* eye exams: one to every SM just after accession to establish baseline diagnostic measures; and then others administered periodically at three-, five-, or eight-year intervals. These periodicities were determined in consultation with SMEs to coincide with existing policies for cognitive assessment for SMs for three and five years. An eight-year interval was also explored to provide increased resolution on the sensitivity of our model outcomes to the periodicity of the comprehensive eye exam.

Under the comprehensive eye exam policies, SMs who self-report a vision problem receive a comprehensive eye examination before progressing to the next year. Self-reporting can occur at the entry stage or during active years. However, the yearly probability of spontaneous self-reporting for SMs with an OVD is assumed to be low, per SME consultation—at most, 5 percent. While the spontaneous self-reporting rate may be smaller than 5 percent, its inclusion in the model provides a more realistic representation of the complexities involved in vision screening for SMs and, by varying this parameter, we determined it had a small impact on our model outcomes.

SMs who are diagnosed with an OVD enter a structured treatment plan, and their vision condition is monitored annually with additional comprehensive eye exams. The success of their yearly treatment for the specific diagnosed OVD is then simulated. We now turn to showing our assumed parameter values for this model.

General Model Inputs and Parameter Values

Inputs to the model are important drivers of the outcomes of the simulation and our recommendations. Although we have discussed the *structure* of the model thus far in this chapter, we now turn to reviewing the specific inputs in the model and the sources we drew on to inform their selection. Table 2.2 summarizes these variables.

The approach to obtaining inputs to the parameters needed for the simulation included three sources: literature reviews, data analysis, and SME opinions. Our SMEs included staff from the Vision Center of Excellence and the Tri-Service Vision Conservation & Readiness Program. In the ideal cases, we had all three sources to help provide ranges for the data, but in many of the cases we had only one or two to draw on for the most accurate, relevant, and up-to-date inputs. This section focuses on the most important inputs; the remaining, less influential, inputs are discussed in Appendix D.

The estimates for the input parameters, such as the prevalence of eye conditions, treatment efficacy, treatment sensitivity, and treatment specificity, have been obtained from the health services literature. We extracted most of the articles from the PubMed database by using a set of search terms ("prevalence of . . .", "efficacy of . . .", "sensitivity and specificity of . . .") followed by the exact name of each category of eye conditions. The studies reviewed for this report use data from various age groups and different countries, including the United States. However, we focus on studies that provide estimates relevant to the population of U.S. adults ages 18 to 29, ideally from studies of that specific population, or, if necessary (and noted in Appendix D), young adult populations from other countries. The inputs for the prevalence of RE, dry eye, glaucoma, and VDTBI come from the U.S. data.

Table 2.2. Key Modeling Parameters and Their Uses

Input	Description and Use	Component
Rate of VDTBI risk factor (TBI)	We probabilistically sample SMs across rates of undiagnosed TBIs	Informs the risk of developing the OVDs over time and the risk of having the OVDs at entry
Rate at which VDTBI occurs with TBI	We probabilistically sample SMs with the OVD conditional on TBIs	
General incidence of OVD	We probabilistically sample SMs according to incidence range of seven OVDs	
Exam sensitivity	We model screening and the true positive rate of detecting the OVD	Informs the performance and accuracy of the exam policies
Exam specificity	We model screening and the true negative rate of detecting the OVD	
Treatment effectiveness	SMs diagnosed with the OVD are put on treatment	Informs the likelihood that treatment is effective
	Treatment outcomes depend on effectiveness; effectiveness decreases with age	
Costs of comprehensive eye exams	We assume a range of costs based on current TRICARE and purchased care exam costs, both initially and for follow-up screenings after treatment	Informs the actual costs of running these exams
Treatment costs	We draw on a range of TRICARE and purchased care costs	
Leave costs	Diagnosis and treatment leads to medical leave	
Attrition	We assume that absent comprehensive eye exams, SMs with undiagnosed OVDs separate at the same rates, with the same patterns across categories of attrition, as an SM average	Informs our modeled rates of separation and costs if treatment fails or OVD goes undiagnosed
Discharge costs	If treatment is ineffective, we assume the SM is medically separated with a onetime medical severance pay	
Replacement costs	We apply recruiting and training costs if an SM is discharged due to ineffective OVD treatment	
Visual readiness value	For each year of service with no OVD, SMs contribute a full visual readiness value based on enlisted or officer pay trajectories	Informs our modeled benefits of diagnosing and treating OVDs
Impact on visual readiness value	An undiagnosed OVD reduces visual readiness value by either a 50% reduction (mild), 100% reduction (moderate), or 150% reduction (severe)	

We extracted multiple estimates for each input parameter from the literature. For instance, there were ten relevant studies available for the prevalence of RE and eight for corneal dystrophies. We then generated summary statistics such as minimum, maximum, mean, and median to inform the simulation model.[1]

Although these incidence and prevalence estimates were based on population averages, additional inputs were included in the model to account for the changes in this risk based on experiencing a TBI or concussion. Of all of the possible OVDs that can occur due to TBI, we focus on VDTBI because of its prevalence and distinctness from the other considered conditions.

Survival or Nonincidence Models

We model incidence using parametric survival curve functions, where *survival* refers to the fraction of SMs who *do not* experience the onset of an OVD. More specifically, these survival functions, denoted as $S(a)$, represent the probability that an SM who enters the military at age 18 without the OVD will not develop the OVD by age a. By definition, $S(a)$ is 100 percent at age 18, since SMs who are not fit do not access. The shape of the function $S(a)$ determines the hazard rate $\lambda(a)$, which indicates the yearly probability of developing the OVD at age a. In our discrete-time model, the yearly hazard rate is given by

$$\lambda(a) = -\Delta S(a)/S(a),$$

where

$$\Delta S(a) = S(a + 1) - S(a).$$

Before running our simulation model, for each OVD (and associated TBI and VDTBI rates for that specific OVD) we precompute the value of $S(a)$ and $\lambda(a)$ for all ages a starting at age 18 and ending at age 60. These presimulation computations allow us to organize the hazard rate by age for each OVD in a lookup table for ease of access. Our simulation model reads the precomputed hazard rate, by age for each OVD and associated RF contained in the lookup table, to probabilistically sample events whereby the SMs acquired the OVDs or associated RFs.

Because there are no representative data that would allow for an accurate estimate of the hazard rate for every OVD for every age for all SMs (given that OVDs can go undiagnosed absent universal comprehensive eye exams), we apply functional form assumptions for $S(a)$. Our model allows the user to choose between two parametric functions: exponential and sigmoid. Our sigmoid survival function takes the lognormal parametric form and, together with the exponential survival function, is one of the standard parametric survival models for actuarial use.[2] We respectively denote our two survival functions as $S_{\exp}(a)$ and $S_{\text{sig}}(a)$. The exponential decay assumes a constant hazard rate $\lambda_{\text{sig}}(a)$, which therefore is independent of age. This type of survival function only requires one input parameter to

---

[1] We use these parameters to generate distributions from which to simulate our SMs, assuming a uniform or generalized triangular distribution of values based on these parameters. When not using the uniform distribution for sampling, we utilize the beta PERT distribution, a continuous probability distribution. This distribution generalizes the triangular distribution and provides increased flexibility in representing uncertainty, enabling the creation of flatter or more peaked distributions compared with the triangular distribution.

[2] Richards, 2012.

define its profile, which is the proportion of SMs who reach the reference final deployable age of 40 without developing the OVD (i.e., $S_{exp}(a)$ when $a = 40$), out of a cohort of SMs who at age 18 do not have the OVD. On the other hand, the sigmoid function assumes low hazard rates at early ages, gradually increasing and peaking at a specific age before gradually decreasing back to lower values for older ages. Mathematically, our sigmoid survival model is given by the complement of the cumulative distribution function of a lognormal probability distribution. Specifying the survival model $S_{sig}(a)$ using a sigmoid function requires one additional input compared with the exponential model—namely, the age $a_{1/2}$ when survival is halfway between 100 percent (i.e., $S_{sig}(0)$) and the final age survival proportion $S_{sig}(40)$, and equal to $(1 + S_{sig}(40))/2$.

Figure 2.1 shows examples of our two survival curves. In these examples, we have chosen both $S_{exp}(40)$ and $S_{sig}(40)$ inputs to be the same value and equal to 70 percent. This value means that in both models, 30 percent of a cohort of SMs who do not have the OVD at entry are expected to have acquired the OVD by age 40.

Figure 2.1. Illustrative Plot of Exponential Survival Curves for a VDTBI by Whether Service Member Has a Diagnosed Traumatic Brain Injury

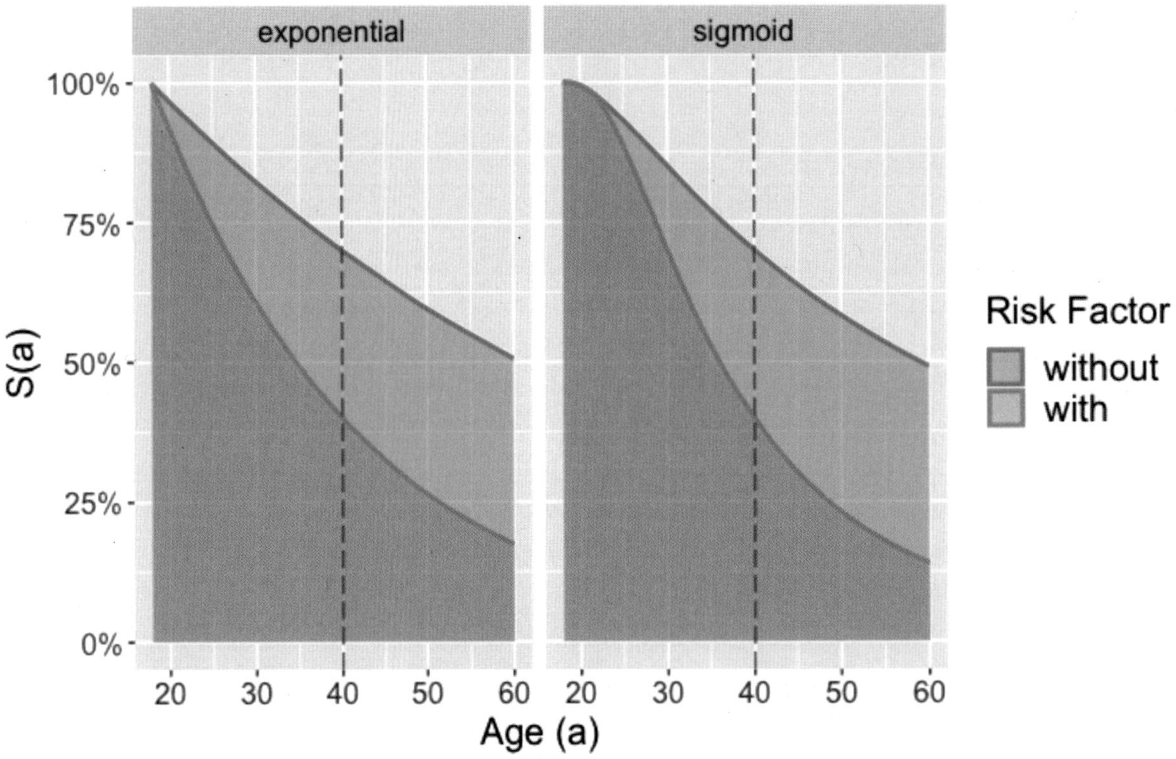

NOTE: In this example, the $S_{exp}(40)$ and $S_{sig}(40)$ input values are both set to 70 percent, and $a_{1/2}$ is 30 years. The odds ratio input value is set to 2 and hence, acquiring VDTBI by age 40 is approximately twice as likely for SMs who have had a TBI, the RF under consideration, by age 18 than those who have not.

This proportion is unrealistically large, but it is used in the figure for the purpose of illustration to better show the differences in the two survival curves. In addition, the age $a_{1/2}$, when the sigmoid model gives a survival proportion of 85 percent (i.e., midway between 70 percent and 100 percent), was chosen to be 30. Generating a look-up table of $S_{exp}(a)$ and $S_{sig}(a)$ for each age ranging from 18 to 60 and using these inputs allows us to plot the two-survival curve in this example.

As mentioned earlier, the only OVD considered in our model that has an associated RF is VDTBI, where the RF is in this case having ever had at least one TBI. For SMs who have had TBIs, we assume they have a higher probability of acquiring VDTBIs compared with those who have never experienced TBIs. The survival curve assumed for SMs with the RF is determined by an input specifying the risk ratio of developing VDTBIs by age 40 relative to SMs without the RF. To provide a clearer understanding, consider an example with a risk ratio value of 2. This means that the survival curves for VDTBI show that, by age 40, the risk of an SM who has suffered at least one concussion by age 18 to acquire a VDTBI is twice that of an SM who has never experienced a concussion. In Figure 2.1, we have example plots of the exponential and sigmoid survival curves, comparing the survival rates of SMs with and without the RF using a risk ratio value of 2. These plots demonstrate the diverging trends in survival rates over time for the two groups.

SMs who never had a TBI by age 18 may still suffer from a TBI during service. Our model assumes a constant hazard rate for TBIs for deployable SMs by YOS. Thus, the survival curve for the TBI RF follows an exponential form. SMs that suffer from the first TBI between the ages of 18 and 40 abruptly transition from following the VDTBI survival curve for those without the RF to the survival curve with the RF. Note that the TBI RF is absorbing; that is to say that this RF is assumed to be irreversible. One can get treated for a TBI, but we assume the acquired additional risk of developing a VDTBI permanently increases once one has suffered from a TBI in their lifetime.

Informing the Survival Function

The literature review informed the prevalence and survival (or the likelihood that an SM *does not* acquire an OVD by a certain age) parameters by condition used in the model. Since many of the values in the literature were prevalence for all levels of severity, we consulted SMEs to identify the relevant articles in the literature to account for (1) severities that are high enough such that it is not plausible for the conditions to go undiagnosed among SMs and (2) their observed differences in the SM population. Table 2.3 includes the inputs for the probability that an SM has the condition by age 18 and the probability of an SM developing the condition by age 40. All inputs for prevalence and survival were sampled using a uniform distribution.

Table 2.3. Prevalence of Condition by Age

Condition/OVD	Probability of Developing OVD by Age 18		Nonprevalence by Age 40	
	Lower Bound	Upper Bound	Lower Bound	Upper Bound
Corneal dystrophy	0.09%	0.13%	99.7%	99.9%
Dry eye	2.03%	5.74%	93.2%	99.9%
Glaucoma	0.16%	0.69%	98.0%	99.5%

Condition/OVD	Probability of Developing OVD by Age 18		Nonprevalence by Age 40	
	Lower Bound	Upper Bound	Lower Bound	Upper Bound
Keratoconus	0.12%	0.90%	99.0%	99.9%
RE	15.0%	50.00%	35%	68.0%
Retinal dystrophy	0.00%	0.14%	99.5%	99.9%
VDTBI	2.30%	8.30%	76.5%	94.4%
			RF Odds Ratio	
VDTBI w/RF	23.0%	66.0%	1.58	3.3

NOTE: See Table D.1 for more detail.

Treatment Inputs

We now turn to our inputs for the assumed efficacy of treatment once an OVD is diagnosed. The literature provided overall treatment efficacy, but given the annual step of our model, we required annual treatment efficacy as well. The calculation we performed to convert the treatment efficacy rates found in literature to an annual treatment efficacy is described here.

Treatment efficacy inputs are as follows:

- Y: treatment efficacy
- a: average years treated with condition
- T: annual treatment efficacy.

Thus,

$$Y = T^a.$$

A factor, c, was used on populations over age 35 to account for the reduction in efficacy of treatments. For the older $T = Y^{\left(\frac{1}{a}\right)}$,

$$T = c \cdot Y^{\left(\frac{1}{a}\right)}.$$

Table 2.4 contains the input values for the end and annual treatment efficacies. Input from the Vision Center of Excellence's SMEs modified the upper values of RE from the civilian literature to account for the high success of treatment to bring SMs to full visual readiness. All inputs in this table were sampled using a uniform distribution. The final row of the table shows how we model the decline in the efficacy of treatment once an SM reaches age 35.

Table 2.4. Treatment Efficacy by Condition

Condition/OVD	Treatment End Efficacy		Treatment Annual Efficacy	
	Lower Bound	Upper Bound	Lower Bound	Upper Bound
Corneal dystrophy	14%	100%	89%	100%
Dry eye	21%	90%	91%	99%
Glaucoma	35%	93%	94%	100%

Condition/OVD	Treatment End Efficacy		Treatment Annual Efficacy	
	Lower Bound	Upper Bound	Lower Bound	Upper Bound
Keratoconus	2%	90%	78%	99%
RE	39%	100%	95%	100%
Retinal dystrophy	31%	71%	93%	98%
VDTBI	4%	92%	83%	100%
Reduction in treatment efficacy by age	15%	25%		

NOTE: See Table D.2 for more detail.

The annual costs, which are the average amounts needed to treat an SM with a diagnosed OVD, are shown in Table 2.5. These costs were sampled as a uniform distribution for all conditions excluding retinal dystrophy, which was sampled from a PERT distribution. For the uniform distribution, the sampling parameters were the lower and upper values; for the PERT distribution, it was the lower, and upper (mode).

Table 2.5. Annual Treatment Costs by Condition

Condition	Yearly Treatment Cost	
	Lower	Upper (Mode)
Corneal dystrophy	$1,765	$1,988
Dry eye	$78	$200
Glaucoma	$640	$930
Keratoconus	$115	$2,150
RE	$50	$263
Retinal dystrophy	$725	$42,500 ($2,000)
VDTBI	$250	$757

NOTE: See Table D.3 for more detail on sources and the set of treatments for each condition.

Performance and Accuracy Inputs of Screening and Comprehensive Eye Exams

The current policy of basic acuity screening only tests for RE and does not provide diagnoses for the other six conditions. The sensitivity and specificity for the basic acuity screening is shown in Table 2.6. The inputs are based on literature review and expert opinion from SMEs from the Vision Center of Excellence. Some sensitivities and specificities (noted in Table 2.7) were modified from the literature review values to account for (1) severities that are high enough to cause the SM to not be deployable and (2) their observed differences in the SM population.

Table 2.6. Accuracy of Basic Acuity Screening

	Sensitivity		Specificity	
Baseline Visual Acuity Screening	**Lower Bound**	**Upper Bound**	**Lower Bound**	**Upper Bound**
RE	38%	98%	58%	98%

The proposed comprehensive eye exam tests for all seven conditions. The sensitivity and specificity of the comprehensive eye exam for each condition is in Table 2.7. The inputs are based on literature review. Uniform sampling is used for these inputs.

Table 2.7. Accuracy of Comprehensive Eye Exams

	Sensitivity		Specificity	
Condition	**Lower Bound**	**Upper Bound**	**Lower Bound**	**Upper Bound**
Corneal dystrophy	63%	94%	73%	98%
Dry eye	63%	98%	70%	98%
Glaucoma	74%	93%	70%	86%
Keratoconus	68%	100%	68%	98%
RE	70%	98%	70%	98%
Retinal dystrophy	82%	100%	67%	98%
VDTBI	78%	89%	95%	98%

NOTE: See Table D.4 for more detail.

Other Fixed Costs

The examination costs and SM replacement costs (including recruiting and training a new SM) in the model are shown in Table 2.8. The costs are fixed and do not change with the age of the SM. These costs are sampled using a uniform distribution, and the inputs were based on our literature review. SMs diagnosed with one or more OVDs undergo yearly follow-up surveillance tests, which have an average cost of $50 per SM per year according to costs provided from the Vision Center of Excellence. These tests assess whether treatment continues to be effective across all diagnosed OVDs. Diagnosed SMs follow a structured treatment plan and continue to receive treatment each year until there is a treatment failure or they otherwise separate from service. The model accounts for a yearly OVD-specific treatment cost incurred by SMs receiving treatment. When an SM is diagnosed with an OVD, we assume that they take a short medical leave of five days. In the year of a treatment failure, a longer medical leave of 20 days is assumed; values for both were provided by the Vision Center of Excellence.

16

Table 2.8. Unit Screening Costs

Cost	Lower	Upper
Basic screening	$27	$33
Comprehensive eye exam	$135	$165
Follow-up exam	$45	$55
Daily medical leave	$180	$220
Replacement	$67,332	$82,294

SOURCES: Replacement costs are from Z. D. Merritt, E. C. McNally, C. S. Allen, C. E. Bruff, G. A. Coleman, K. N. Harms, G. M. Mallie, C. W. Perdue, S. R. Putansu, T. L. Richardson, et al., *Military Personnel: Personnel and Cost Data Associated with Implementing DoD's Homosexual Conduct Policy*, Government Accountability Office, GAO-11-170, 2011, updated to 2022 dollars with Consumer Price Index for Urban Consumers. Other costs are based on TRICARE data or direct estimates from Vision Center of Excellence SMEs.

Visual Readiness Value and the Readiness Cost of Ocular and Visual Dysfunction

A crucial aspect of the simulation model focuses on tracking the costs associated with lost productivity and the impact that undiagnosed OVDs has on readiness. The model operates under the assumption that each SM contributes a *visual readiness value*, which is influenced by their level of experience and whether they have full visual fitness. In the model, SMs are deemed to have visual fitness if they are free from any OVD or if they are receiving effective treatment for all OVDs they may have. Having an OVD that is treated effectively is assumed to impose no limitations on SMs' duties and tasks and consequently does not diminish their visual readiness. On the other hand, SMs who have at least one undiagnosed OVD, or who have been diagnosed with at least one OVD but the treatment has proven ineffective, are considered to have reduced visual readiness. The primary benefit of comprehensive eye exams is thus to diagnose otherwise undiagnosed OVDs and treat them, restoring the SM to full visual fitness. We focus on visual fitness because we assume that other medical conditions are accounted for in our measure of all-other-cause attrition discussed above.

The readiness value of an SM with full vision fitness can be assumed to have a yearly value that starts at a certain level at age 18, growing with experience and pay grade, and then stabilizes at a constant value. We express this yearly readiness value as a function of age (a) using the following equation:

$$v_{fit}(a) = v_{fit}^*[b + (1 - b)(1 - e^{-\rho a})].$$

Here, b is a value between zero and 1 that determines the age dependency of the readiness value, and ρ characterizes the rate at which SMs gain experience and reach their expected value in terms of their ability and contribution to readiness. If b is set to 1, then $v_{fit}(a)$ becomes independent of age, implying that the value of an SM with full vision fitness at age 18 is the same as at any older age. On the other hand, if b is set to zero, $v_{fit}(a)$ becomes age-dependent and increases rapidly from a value of zero at age 18 to a value that approaches v_{fit}^* at age 40. For values of b between zero and 1, $v_{fit}(a)$ varies with age and exhibits a rapid increase from a nonzero value of bv_{fit}^* at age 18 to a value that approaches v_{fit}^* at age 40. To simplify the interpretation of model input parameters, instead of directly specifying the value of parameter b, we provide the starting dollar amount of readiness for an eighteen-year-old SM ($v_{fit}(18)$), and then calculate b from $v_{fit}(18)/v_{fit}^*$. By using this formulation, we can model the readiness value of SMs with full vision fitness, accounting for age-related variations and the rate at which experience accumulates.

In a similar manner, we take into account the reduced value of visual readiness contributed by SMs who have an undiagnosed OVD. We assume that this value, denoted as $v_{unfit}(a)$, is dependent on age (a) and is proportional to $v_{fit}(a)$. Hence, it can be expressed as $v_{unfit}(a) = \kappa v_{fit}(a)$, where the parameter κ is a proportionality constant ranging from −1 to 1, representing the reduction in visual readiness resulting from an undiagnosed OVD.

A positive κ value that is lower than 1 indicates a partial reduction to the SM's contribution to force readiness; that is, an SM with an undiagnosed OVD still can perform at least some of their duties, albeit in a limited capacity. On the other hand, if the κ value is equal to zero, it implies that an SM with an undiagnosed OVD provides no contribution to total force readiness, similar to not having the SM serve at all. Finally, a negative κ value suggests that an SM with an undiagnosed OVD has a detrimental impact on total force readiness beyond merely the lack of an SM in that position. This implies that the individual's OVD causes active harm to the force.

The plots shown in Figure 2.2 illustrate two examples where we have set $v_{fit}^* = \$50K$, $v_{fit}(18) = \$20K$, and $\rho = 0.5$. The plot to the left illustrates an example where the parameter κ is

Figure 2.2. Illustrative Plot Depicting the Readiness Value as a Function of Age for Two Examples of Kappa Value

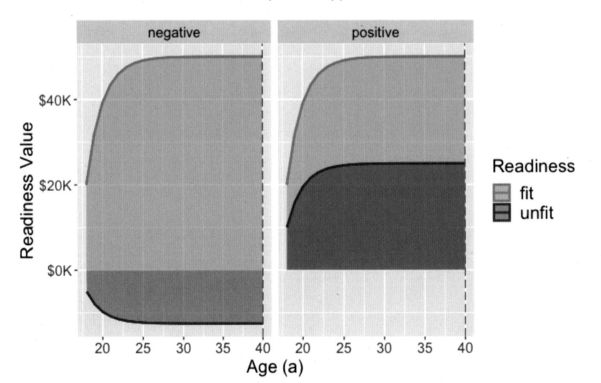

NOTE: Our first example to the left considers a κ value that is negative, thereby leading to the SM subtracting readiness value from the total force for every year in which the red region is under $0, while that to the right considers a positive κ value, whereby the SM is still contributing a positive value, but at a reduced rate.

negative and equal to $\kappa = -0.25$, while the plot to the right illustrates the case where κ is positive and equal to $\kappa = 0.5$. The plot shows how the visual readiness values at each age of deployable SM with full vision fitness (green) and deployable SMs with an undiagnosed OVD who are not visually fit (red).

Let us now consider a scenario where an SM remains visually fit until age a_{VD}, at which point they acquire an undiagnosed OVD but continue to serve until age 40. The overall visual readiness value of this SM is determined by summing the $v_{fit}(a)$ contributions from ages 18 to a_{VD}, and the $v_{unfit}(a)$ contributions from ages a_{VD} to 40. Thus, the cumulative value on readiness is given by

$$V(a_{VD}) = \sum_{a=18}^{a_{VD}-1} v_{fit}(a) + \sum_{a=a_{VD}}^{40} v_{unfit}(a).$$

This equation can be reexpressed as

$$V(a_{VD}) = \left[V_{fit}(18) - V_{fit}(a_{VD})\right] + V_{unfit}(a_{VD}),$$

by introducing two cumulative quantities, defined as follows:

1. $V_{fit}(a_{VD})$ is the cumulative value of an SM being visual fit between ages a_{VD} and 40, which is given by

$$V_{fit}(a_{VD}) = \sum_{a=a_{VD}}^{40} v_{fit}(a),$$

2. $V_{unfit}(a_{VD})$ is the cumulative value of an SM having an undiagnosed OVD between ages a_{VD} and 40, which is given by

$$V_{unfit}(a_{VD}) = \sum_{a=a_{VD}}^{40} v_{unfit}(a).$$

Consider the case where an SM develops an OVD at age a_{VD} and is diagnosed with having the OVD at age $a_D > a_{VD}$. For the sake of argument, assume in this case that when the SM is diagnosed with having the OVD, the severity of the OVD is advanced and the condition cannot be treated, resulting in the SM being discharged. Under this scenario, the cumulative value on readiness is given by

$$V(a_{VD}, a_D) = \sum_{a=18}^{a_{VD}-1} v_{fit}(a) + \sum_{a=a_{VD}}^{a_D-1} v_{unfit}(a).$$

Figure 2.3 illustrates an example for this type of case where we have set $a_{VD} = 25$ and $a_D = 35$, and for a positive κ value. The readiness value is $V(a_{VD}, a_D)$ is illustrated in the plot as the sum of the green area when the deployable SM has vision fitness and the sum of the red area when the SM acquires an OVD that is not diagnosed and thus has reduced visual readiness. At age 35, the SM is diagnosed with an untreatable OVD and is discharged. In this example (but not in our model), the SM is not replaced by another SM at age 35.

Figure 2.3. Illustrative Plot Showing the Readiness Value as a Function of Age

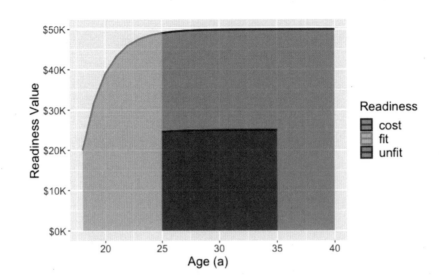

NOTE: This illustrative plot shows the readiness value as a function of age for an example trajectory of an SM who develops an OVD at age 25 and is discharged from deployable active duty at age 35 after being diagnosed with the OVD, which in this case is assumed to be untreatable. In this example, we assume a positive κ value. The accrued readiness value of this SM is given by the sum of the green and the red areas. The cost to readiness is shown by the blue area.

The cost to readiness is then computed by finding the difference between the readiness of a similar SM who retains vision fitness to age 40 minus the accrued readiness value $V(a_{VD}, a_D)$ of the SM who acquired an OVD at age a_{VD} and was diagnosed and discharged at age a_D. In this case, the cost to readiness can be expressed as

$$C(a_{VD}, a_D) = \sum_{a=a_{VD}}^{a_D-1} [v_{fit}(a) - v_{unfit}(a)] + \sum_{a=a_D}^{40} v_{fit}(a).$$

For our example, shown in Figure 2.3, the readiness cost is illustrated in the plot as the sum of the blue area. For the case where the discharged SM is replaced, the simulation model takes into account the cost for the replacement and reduces the readiness cost by removing the second term that enters the equation describing $C(a_{VD}, a_D)$. This is because the replacement is assumed to have full vision fitness and retains it to age 40, hence compensating for the loss in readiness of the discharged SM.

The example we considered provides a simple illustration of how readiness cost due to undiagnosed OVD is calculated. In our simple example above, we assumed that the SM is diagnosed with an untreatable OVD and is discharged. We now consider the case when at the age of diagnosis, a_D, the SM enters treatment and returns to having full visual fitness. During the years when treatment is effective, the SM does not contribute to readiness cost, while if the treatment is ineffective, the SM is immediately discharged with a medical severance payment. If we denote the age of treatment failure as a_F, then the readiness value $V(a_{VD}, a_D, a_F)$ and the readiness cost $C(a_{VD}, a_D, a_F)$ for this case is respectively computed as

$$V(a_{VD}, a_D, a_F) = \sum_{a=18}^{a_{VD}-1} v_{fit}(a) + \sum_{a=a_{VD}}^{a_D-1} v_{unfit}(a) + \sum_{a=a_D}^{a_F-1} v_{fit}(a) + I_R(a_F) \sum_{a=a_F}^{40} v_{fit}(a),$$

$$C(a_{VD}, a_D, a_F) = \sum_{a=a_{VD}}^{a_D-1} (v_{fit}(a) - v_{unfit}(a)) + (1 - I_R(a_F)) \sum_{a=a_F+1}^{40} v_{fit}(a).$$

Here, $I_R(a_F)$ is an indicator function that is equal to one if $a_F < 40$ and treatment failure of SMs leads to a replacement of the SM and is equal to zero otherwise. The indicator function removes the second term when we are considering replacement of SMs who cannot be treated for their OVDs.

Our model implementation calculates the readiness cost in a more practical manner, avoiding the complexities involved in the formal equations presented in this section. It keeps track of the vision fitness status of each SM and maintains a continuous tally of accrued readiness. When an SM retires or is discharged prematurely from active duty, the accumulated readiness value is subtracted from the maximum possible value. The maximum value is determined by summing the vision fitness $v_{fit}(a)$ scores from age 18 to either age 40 or the chosen retirement age from active duty—whichever is greater.

As mentioned previously, the value of a ready year is given by v_{fit}^*, and it represents the yearly readiness value of an SM with full vision fitness. We can use our computed readiness value of an SM to calculate the total number of years they operated at full readiness. The effective number of visual readiness years is then obtained by dividing $V(a_{VD}, a_D, a_F)$ by v_{fit}^*. This effective number of visual readiness years takes into account the additional visual readiness years provided by a replacement, should one be needed.

Informing the Visual Readiness Value Function

Yearly visual readiness values were estimated based on calculating Regular Military Compensation (RMC), which is the sum of monthly pay, housing allowances, and subsistence allowances by pay grade, for both enlisted SMs and officers. These are shown in Table 2.9. This compensation was drawn from the January 2023 DoD Office of the Under Secretary of Defense for Personnel and Readiness (OUSD[P&R]) *Green Book*, which contains all of the components necessary to calculate RMC for any given enlisted or officer pay grade in its Tables A2 and A3. We then assumed that a given SM rises through pay grades, matching the pay grade of the median of the distribution of SMs in a given pay grade, as shown in the *Green Book's* Table A6, "Military Personnel by Pay Cell" and checked to ensure that this rate was no faster than statutorily allowed given time-in-service and time-in-rate requirements.[3] The RMC of an SM by YOS is shown below, as is the corresponding pay grade.

---

[3] DoD, OUSD(P&R), Directorate of Compensation, *Selected Military Compensation Tables [Green Book]*, January 1, 2023.

For modeling purposes, we opted to smooth this set of discrete points with continuous functions shown in Figure 2.4. Fitting the data to our function form, we can extract key model inputs regarding our smoothed function that provides the visual readiness values by age, shown in Table 2.10.

Table 2.9. Readiness Value Based on Annual Regular Military Compensation by Years of Service and Enlisted or Officer Status, in 2022 Dollars

YOS	Enlisted	Pay Grade	YOS	Officer	Pay Grade
0	48,058.56	E1/E2	0	68,487.00	O1
1	51,957.12	E3	1	68,487.00	O1
2	54,675.42	E3/E4	2	84,799.32	O2
3	57,397.32	E4	3	93,489.72	O2
4	59,085.72	E4	4	109,028.40	O3
5	59,085.72	E4	5	109,028.40	O3
6	68,766.12	E5	6	112,754.40	O3
7	68,766.12	E5	7	112,754.40	O3
8	71,581.32	E5	8	116,836.80	O3
9	71,581.32	E5	9	116,836.80	O3
10	78,761.28	E6	10	133,959.60	O4
11	78,761.28	E6	11	133,959.60	O4
12	81,749.28	E6	12	138,888.00	O4
13	81,749.28	E6	13	138,888.00	O4
14	82,663.68	E6	14	142,315.20	O4
15	82,663.68	E6	15	142,315.20	O4
16	92,905.68	E7	16	155,950.80	O5
17	92,905.68	E7	17	155,950.80	O5
18	94,763.28	E7	18	159,342.00	O5
19	94,763.28	E7	19	159,342.00	O5
20	95,479.68	E7	20	162,693.60	O5
21	95,479.68	E7	21	162,693.60	O5
22	97,895.28	E7	22	166,498.80	O5

SOURCE: DoD, OUSD(P&R), Directorate of Compensation, 2023.

Figure 2.4. Smoothed Function of Readiness Values

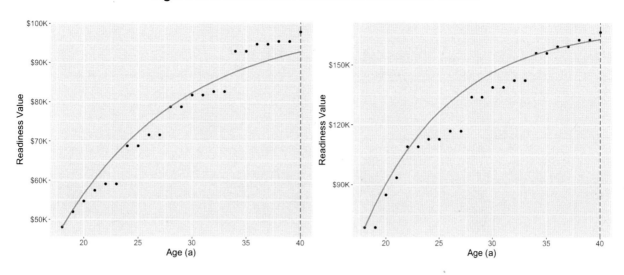

Table 2.10. Parameters from Smoothed Function of Readiness Values

SM	v^*_{fit}	b	ρ
Enlisted	$100,000	0.48	0.09
Officers	$170,000	0.40	0.01215

Following Krull and colleagues, 2019,[4] discharge costs are based on the medical separation payment due, assuming that the previously undiagnosed OVD would not result in a disability rating of 30 percent or higher. Thus, these costs rise with YOS and are calculated as the product of YOS and base monthly pay times two. We use the three-year minimum for YOS, given the assumption that a combat-related OVD would be detected under the baseline screening policy. See Table 2.11 for these costs.

As discussed above, we assume under all scenarios that status quo all-cause attrition rates from the military remain unchanged (i.e., that undiagnosed OVD is not correlated with other forms of disability or types of separation). We calculate these rates based on DoD's *Valuation of the Medicare-Eligible Retiree Health Care Fund* report from January 2022, which reports discharge rates by type.[5] We sum rates for each year of service separately across enlisted SMs and officers across: death rates (Table F2 in the DoD report), retirement rates (Tables F3 and F4), and withdrawal rates (Tables F5

---

[4] Heather Krull, Philip Armour, Kathryn A. Edwards, Kristin Van Abel, Linda Cottrell, and Gulrez Shah Azhar, "The Relationship Between Disability Evaluation and Accession Medical Standards," Santa Monica, Calif.: RAND Corporation, 2019.

[5] DoD, Office of the Actuary, 2022.

Table 2.11. Medical Severance Pay for Discharged Service Members by Years of Service (YOS) and Enlisted or Officer Status, in 2022 Dollars

YOS	Enlisted	Pay Grade	YOS	Officer	Pay Grade
0	12,200.40	E1/E2	0	21,823.20	O1
1	13,559.40	E3	1	21,823.20	O1
2	15,101.10	E3/E4	2	28,636.20	O2
3	16,644.60	E4	3	32,981.40	O2
4	23,318.40	E4	4	51,758.40	O3
5	29,148.00	E4	5	64,698.00	O3
6	41,086.80	E5	6	81,363.60	O3
7	47,934.60	E5	7	94,924.20	O3
8	58,536.00	E5	8	113,928.00	O3
9	65,853.00	E5	9	128,169.00	O3
10	83,418.00	E6	10	165,096.00	O4
11	91,759.80	E6	11	181,605.60	O4
12	106,077.60	E6	12	207,972.00	O4
13	114,917.40	E6	13	225,303.00	O4
14	125,890.80	E6	14	250,630.80	O4
15	134,883.00	E6	15	268,533.00	O4
16	168,278.40	E7	16	319,449.60	O5
17	178,795.80	E7	17	339,415.20	O5
18	194,886.00	E7	18	369,554.40	O5
19	205,713.00	E7	19	390,085.20	O5
20	0	E7	20	0	O5
21	0	E7	21	0	O5
22	0	E7	22	0	O5

NOTE: Figures calculated using disability severance pay formula applied to pay from Table 2.9.

and F6). These rates are combined with our age-specific lookup table containing presimulation computations of the survival and hazard rates. Our simulation model reads the all-other-cause attrition contained in the lookup table to probabilistically sample events, whereby the SMs leave active deployable duty due to all other non-vision-related causes. The attrition rate for SMs ages 40–60 includes the retirement rate of active duty. All-cause-attrition rates are shown in Table 2.12.

Table 2.12. All-Other-Cause Attrition Rates, by Years of Service (YOS) and Enlisted or Officer Status

YOS	Enlisted	Officer
0	0.074	0.007
1	0.062	0.012
2	0.109	0.031
3	0.282	0.084
4	0.199	0.097
5	0.193	0.078
6	0.123	0.088
7	0.162	0.092
8	0.110	0.073
9	0.101	0.006
10	0.083	0.092
11	0.075	0.072
12	0.063	0.051
13	0.071	0.037
14	0.064	0.028
15	0.032	0.022
16	0.028	0.016
17	0.019	0.012
18	0.011	0.007
19	0.467	0.303
20	0.276	0.183
21	0.245	0.156
22	0.253	0.148
23	0.385	0.156
24	0.263	0.164
25	0.442	0.177
26	0.232	0.176
27	0.198	0.190
28	0.235	0.184
29	0.667	0.383
30	0.585	0.331
31	0.611	0.234
32	0.596	0.233

YOS	Enlisted	Officer
33	0.570	0.273
34	0.605	0.270
35	0.573	0.275
36	0.573	0.279
37	0.573	0.373
38	0.573	0.313
39	0.573	0.513
40	1.000	1.000

SOURCE: DoD, Office of the Actuary, 2022, Tables F2–F6. Each number corresponds to the fraction of service members separating for all other causes in that year of service.

Model Parameter Uncertainties

As can be seen from the above tables, many of the model inputs can fall within a substantial range of plausible values, making it crucial to conduct uncertainty and robustness analyses to assess the effectiveness of different policies under varying plausible scenarios. Additionally, sensitivity analyses play a vital role in quantifying the influence and uncertainty of each parameter on the outcomes of the simulation model. Our simulation model recognizes the presence of significant uncertainty in parameter values, necessitating a comprehensive analysis of uncertainty, robustness, and sensitivity. Through the implementation of Latin hypercube sampling (LHS), we aim to capture the inherent variability and bias in the model inputs.[6] These analyses enable us to evaluate policies under diverse scenarios and quantify the impact of individual parameters on the model outcomes, facilitating informed decisionmaking in the face of uncertainty.

The LHS is an efficient method for creating experimental designs that encompass a wide range of parameter values; it enables the exploration of unique combinations of parameter inputs, capturing the variability and uncertainty inherent in the model. Moreover, by incorporating the beta PERT distribution, we can sample parameter values with a bias toward specific modes, thus reflecting the most likely values within a range. The process of LHS involves dividing each parameter range into intervals and randomly selecting one value from each interval to create a unique combination of parameter values. This approach ensures that each parameter is sampled across its entire range while maintaining the overall distribution and correlation between parameters. By carefully constructing the sampling design, LHS allows for efficient exploration of the parameter space and provides valuable insights into the behavior and performance of the simulation model. Our uncertainty analyses allow us to evaluate the performance and consistency of different policies in the face of uncertain inputs. By quantifying the ranges of uncertainty and assessing the robustness of the model outcomes, we gain

---

[6] R. L. Iman, J. C. Helton, and J. E. Campbell, "An Approach to Sensitivity Analysis of Computer Models: Part I—Introduction, Input Variable Selection and Preliminary Variable Assessment," *Journal of Quality Technology*, Vol. 13, No. 3, October 1981.

valuable insights into which policies are most effective across a spectrum of conditions. Sensitivity analyses complement these efforts by providing a deeper understanding of the leverage and influence that each parameter, along with its associated uncertainty, exerts on the simulation model's results.

Cost-Effectiveness and Cost-Benefit Analyses

Our simulation model generates outputs that include the costs accrued by each SM due to the administration of comprehensive eye exams, treatment costs, possible discharge costs, and replacement costs, as well as the accrued visual readiness value for each SM during their deployable lifetime. We aggregate these outputs to conduct a cost-effectiveness analysis (CEA) to compare different comprehensive eye examination policies regarding their total costs and overall readiness outcomes. CEA is a method that enables decisionmakers to determine the most efficient use of available resources when multiple options are available. It is often used to evaluate policy interventions in health by focusing on a specific outcome measure, such as years of life saved or quality-adjusted life years. In our case, CEA involves assessing the costs associated with comprehensive eye exams and treating SMs who have OVDs and evaluating the impact of these interventions on military readiness. The CEA analysis is performed from the perspective of DoD, using the current policy of basic acuity tests as the comparator policy. This analysis considers both the costs involved in implementing the comprehensive eye exams and treatment programs and the potential benefits or gains in military readiness. The benefit outcome measure we focus on is the readiness years gained (RYG), which is determined by calculating the difference between the expected effective number of readiness years under a specific policy and the number obtained under the reference or comparator policy. In other words, RYG represents the additional years of military readiness gained or lost due to the implementation of a particular comprehensive eye examination policy compared with the current screening policy.

Using the computed RYG of a policy relative to its comparator policy, and the difference between their fixed set of accrued costs, we can calculate a net monetary benefit (NMB) of the policy. By denoting the RYG as ΔY and the accrued cost difference as ΔC_F, the NMB is given by

$$E[NMB] = \lambda \, E[\Delta Y] - E[\Delta C_F],$$

where λ is the willingness to pay for one year of readiness, or the assumed value of a year of readiness to the military. If the expected NMB is positive (i.e., $NMB > 0$), the policy is cost-effective compared with the comparator policy. From our expression of the expected NMB, we have that, for a policy to be cost beneficial,

$$\lambda \leq E[\Delta C_F]/E[\Delta Y].$$

Consequently, we can define the maximum willingness to pay for the policy (λ_{max}) to be cost beneficial by setting the expected NMB to zero, and hence $\lambda_{max} = \frac{E[\Delta C_F]}{E[\Delta Y]}$. Note that the benefits and costs are computed by taking the expectation with respect to the set of model parameters described above and the stochastic model runs. This formulation is analogous to an NMB of medical interventions where effectiveness is measured as quality-adjusted life years gained.[7]

In addition, one can express the benefits ($\lambda \, E[\Delta Y]$) in terms of averted readiness costs, expressing both benefits and costs in the same units of analysis—namely, dollars. This approach allows our results to be interpreted as a CBA for a given λ, translating all costs and benefits to monetary terms. The CBA considers both the financial costs and the monetary value of the outcomes achieved. It involves assigning monetary values to military readiness gains, as well as the costs of comprehensive eye exams, treatment, and potential discharge of SMs.

---

[7] A. A. Stinnett and J. Mullahy, "Net Health Benefits: A New Framework for the Analysis of Uncertainty in Cost-Effectiveness Analysis," *Medical Decision Making*, Vol. 18, No. 2, Suppl., April 1998.

Chapter 3

Cost-Benefit Analysis of Alternative Eye Examination Policies

In this chapter, we present the analyses of the outputs generated by our discrete-time microsimulation model. We provide tables and plots displaying the statistics derived from these outputs. The objective of our model was to simulate the same SM cohort under different OVD screening or examination policies, enabling decisionmakers to compare readiness outcomes and policy costs through CBA. To achieve this, we ran the simulation model under a wide range of parameter values, each sampled within their uncertainty ranges while considering various scenarios on the impacts of undiagnosed OVDs on the force.

By modeling each individual's full set of trajectories, we could examine the impact of different OVD screening or examination policies on readiness and cost throughout SMs' deployable lifetimes. For each case run, we analyzed the trajectories of all SMs and calculated average values for visual readiness, visual readiness cost, total cost, and net monetary benefit. We thus present statistics that illustrate the distribution of these average outcomes across sets of case runs with similar model specifications and assumptions, such as the consideration of varying visual readiness values based on enlisted versus officer compensation and ranges of kappa (κ) values representing the reduction in readiness caused by undiagnosed OVD.

Sensitivity Analysis

Before presenting our policy comparison analyses, we briefly summarize the results of our sensitivity analysis, which is crucial in analyzing the outputs of our microsimulation model. This analysis helps identify the various contributions of inputs, assess model robustness, and evaluate the stability and consistency of outputs across different input variations. As was shown in Chapter 2, there is a wide range of plausible parameter values and assumptions; the sensitivity analysis shows how reliant our results are on each of these values and assumptions, and thus what the most impactful sources of uncertainty are.

During the sensitivity analysis, we varied input values to determine the factors that have the most significant leverage on the outcomes of interest. The leverage of an input variable refers to how sensitive the output values are to changes in that specific input variable. By exploring different parameter values, we gained insights into the impacts of various factors on the model outputs. To quantify leverage and gain insights into the importance of different inputs on the outputs, we calculated Spearman's partial rank correlation coefficient (PRCC) between the model input parameters and the outputs.

29

The PRCC is a valuable measure that considers the influence of other variables, providing a comprehensive understanding of the relationships between model inputs and outputs. It goes beyond simple correlation analysis by accounting for the variability and effects of other model inputs. By using the PRCC, we can obtain a more accurate assessment of the associations between inputs and outputs, even revealing inverse associations that may not be evident through simple correlation.

The plot presented in Figure 3.1 provides a visual representation of the most statistically significant PRCCs between the model inputs and readiness outcomes for illustrative purposes, while the PRCCs for all inputs are shown in Appendix B. This plot allows us to analyze the influence of various parameters on the overall readiness.

Figure 3.1. Sensitivity Analysis of Inputs with a *P*-Value Less Than 0.125

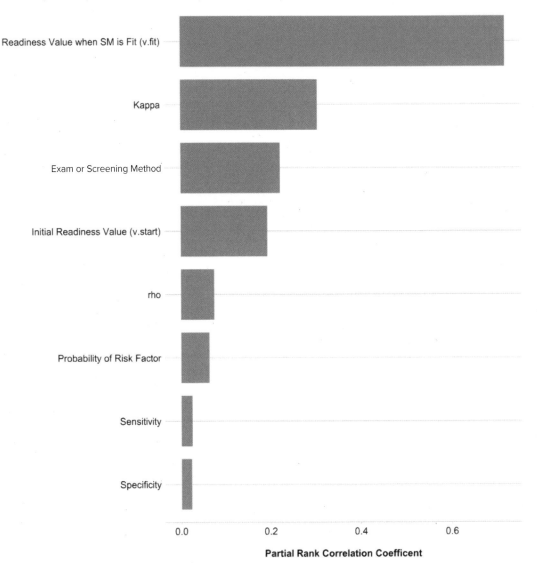

On examining the plot, we observe that several parameters related to how readiness changes with age exhibit a substantial leverage on the overall readiness. "Exam or screening method" refers to whether basic acuity screening or a comprehensive eye exam is chosen as our policy. Specifically, the parameters v_{fit}^*, b, and ρ, shown in Table 2.10, are denoted as v.fit, v.start, and rho, respectively, in the plot. These parameters significantly contribute to the readiness outcomes. Another parameter, κ, labeled as kappa in the plot and corresponding to the reduction in readiness caused by an undiagnosed OVD, also demonstrates considerable leverage on the model output.

Furthermore, it is noteworthy that the probability of having a TBI at age 18 (the probability of risk factor) also exhibits significant leverage on the readiness outcomes. This factor plays a crucial role in influencing readiness levels.

Finally, we observe that the specificity associated with the screening on examination policy holds substantial leverage on the model output. This indicates that the accuracy and precision of the examination policy and its procedures greatly impact readiness outcomes.

In summary, the plot provides valuable insights into the influential parameters and factors that affect readiness outcomes. It highlights the significance of certain parameters related to age-related changes in readiness, as well as the influence of OVD and TBI probabilities and screening specificity. These findings contribute to a better understanding of the model's behavior and assist in making informed decisions regarding readiness improvement strategies.

Given the multidimensionality of all of the modeling inputs and outputs, the insights gained from our sensitivity analysis have informed our approach to presenting the model results. Our selection of visualizations, plots, and tables in the following section are thus intended to effectively communicate the pertinent findings informed by the importance of each parameter input.

The Experimental Design and How Model Outputs Are Presented

There is already considerable uncertainty over readiness value and the readiness cost of undiagnosed OVDs. As such, we do not additionally model these values for specific occupational specialties. This decision was not intended to imply that the same examination policy would be equally cost-effective for all occupational specialties; indeed, the services already vary in their visual requirements and screening policies for specific occupations—most notably, that of pilot. The reader should examine the importance of readiness value and loss associated with OVDs in considering their assumed readiness values for any given occupation.

The readiness loss itself is quantified by the κ parameter. In the outputs presented in this section, we consider simulation models with three different values for κ. We consider a positive value for κ of 0.5, which signifies a mild impact on readiness for undiagnosed SMs, implying that their readiness is equivalent to 50 percent of the readiness provided by a fully visually fit SM. We also considered κ values of zero (which we refer to as a *moderate readiness impact*) and −0.5. (which we refer to as a *severe readiness impact*). A zero κ value indicates zero readiness contribution for undiagnosed SMs relative to visually fit ones. A negative κ value indicates that undiagnosed SMs hinder the overall readiness of a unit.

In this chapter, our analysis focuses on readiness costs, total costs, and the NMB derived from the CBA. The NMB compares readiness cost with total costs to determine the cost-effectiveness of the policy. When presenting the data, we group and display the four policy options (current basic acuity screenings, or comprehensive eye exams with the three periodicities discussed above), examining visual readiness value based on enlisted or officer pay trajectories separately. Furthermore, we highlight the conditions for different κ values within each policy option. We combine box plots and violin plots to visualize the data. The violin plots depict the probability distribution or outcome distribution along the y-axis. In contrast, the box plots represent the median value, interquartile range, and full range of values extending from the minimum to the maximum. In Appendix A, we present the same results shown in the plots as tables in numerical form.

The Readiness Cost of Undiagnosed Ocular and Visual Dysfunctions

Figure 3.2 showcases combined violin and box plots, enabling a separate comparison of the distribution of deployable lifetime readiness costs per SM across four distinct policy options, various assumptions for the value κ, and separate comparisons for the enlisted and officer pay trajectories.

Our analysis reveals that the comprehensive eye examination policy leads to a substantial reduction in readiness costs compared with the baseline screening. As anticipated, the reduction in readiness costs is most notable when κ values are negative (the red violin plots, where OVDs have the most severe impacts on readiness) and when the comprehensive eye exam is conducted at a higher frequency—specifically, every three years. Given the higher readiness values of officers when fit, it is not surprising that the readiness costs of undiagnosed OVDs among officers are substantially higher than among enlisted SMs.

The Role of Exam Specificity on Readiness Value and Readiness Cost

To assess the robustness of our readiness cost results as a function of our assumed screening accuracy, we conducted further analyses by exploring the sensitivity and specificity values associated with the baseline and comprehensive eye exams. Because of the uncertainty over testing accuracy for this population, to cover a range of scenarios we considered both optimistic and pessimistic case scenarios. In the optimistic case scenarios, we used screening accuracy characterized by sensitivity and specificity values sampled from the lowest fiftieth percentile of their uncertainty range. For comprehensive eye exams, we used sensitivity and specificity values sampled from the highest fiftieth percentile of their uncertainty range. In effect, this optimistic scenario assumes that current screening policy is on the less accurate range of plausibility and that comprehensive eye exams are on the more accurate range of plausibility.

Conversely, in the pessimistic case scenarios, we reversed this assumption. Baseline screenings were characterized by sensitivity and specificity values sampled from the highest fiftieth percentile of their uncertainty range, while comprehensive eye exams were defined by sensitivity and specificity values sampled from the lowest fiftieth percentile of their uncertainty range. Figure 3.3 presents combined violin and box plots illustrating the optimistic case scenario, while Figure 3.4 showcases the pessimistic case scenario.

Figure 3.2. Total Readiness Cost per 1,000 Enlisted Service Members of Different Screening or Comprehensive Eye Exam Policies, by Assumed Impact of Undiagnosed Ocular and Visual Dysfunction on Visual Readiness and by Full Readiness Value

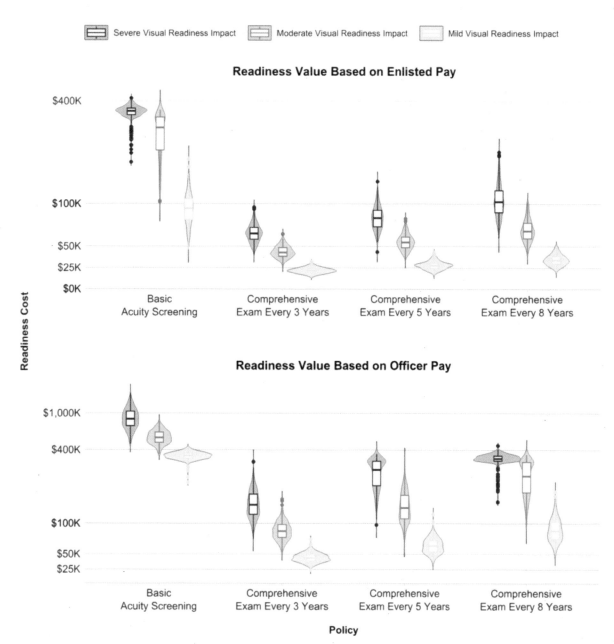

NOTE: Color coding corresponds to the assumed impact of an undiagnosed OVD on visual readiness values. Green corresponds to *mild visual readiness impact* (i.e., where undiagnosed SMs still contribute readiness value, but their contribution is reduced by half); blue to *moderate visual readiness impact* (i.e., where an undiagnosed OVD reduces the visual readiness value contributions of an SM completely to zero); and red to *severe visual readiness impact* (i.e., where an undiagnosed SM subtracts from force readiness by one-half of their fully healthy visual readiness value). The y-axis is the total readiness cost of undiagnosed OVDs across the 1,000 simulated SMs and 300 simulated runs, and hence shows total dollar figures for every 1,000 SMs. Box plots indicate the interquartile range (white rectangle) and median (horizontal line in this rectangle), while violin plots show probability density function based on all runs of each policy frequency and readiness value reduction scenario. We vary the value of full visual readiness illustratively based on either average enlisted or officer pay trajectories.

33

Figure 3.3. Total Readiness Cost per 1,000 Enlisted Service Members of Different Screening or Comprehensive Eye Exam Policies, by Assumed Impact of Undiagnosed Ocular and Visual Dysfunction on Visual Readiness and by Full Readiness Value, Optimistic Screening Scenario Assumed

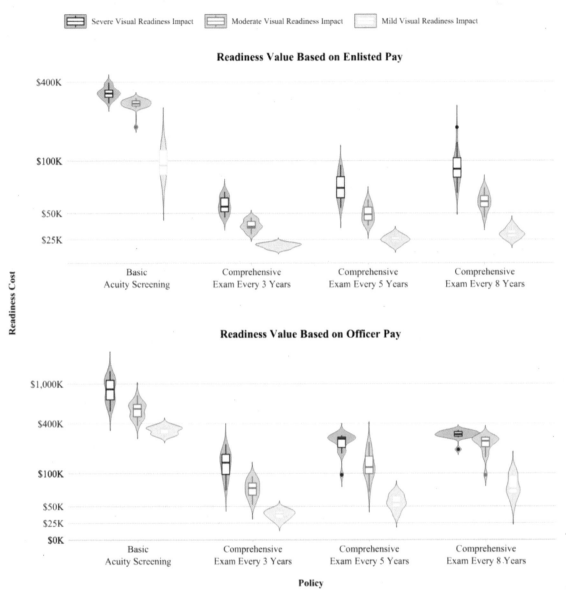

NOTE: Color coding corresponds to the assumed impact of an undiagnosed OVD on visual readiness values. Green corresponds to *mild visual readiness impact* (i.e., where undiagnosed SMs still contribute readiness value, but their contribution is reduced by half); blue to *moderate visual readiness impact* (i.e., where an undiagnosed OVD reduces the visual readiness value contributions of an SM completely to zero); and red to *severe visual readiness impact* (i.e., where an undiagnosed SM subtracts from force readiness by one-half of their fully healthy visual readiness value). The y-axis is the total readiness cost of undiagnosed OVDs across the 1,000 simulated SMs and 300 simulated runs, and hence shows total dollar figures for every 1,000 SMs. Box plots indicate the interquartile range (white rectangle) and median (horizontal line in this rectangle), while violin plots show probability density function based on all runs of each policy frequency and readiness value reduction scenario. We vary the value of full visual readiness illustratively based on either average enlisted or officer pay trajectories. Baseline screening specificity and sensitivity are sampled from the lower half of the previous range, while comprehensive screening specificity and sensitivity are sampled from the higher half of the previous range, thereby assuming an "optimistic" position of comprehensive screening vis-à-vis baseline screening policy.

Figure 3.4. Total Readiness Cost per 1,000 Enlisted Service Members of Different Screening or Comprehensive Eye Exam Policies, by Assumed Impact of Undiagnosed Ocular and Visual Dysfunction on Visual Readiness and by Full Readiness Value, Pessimistic Screening Scenario Assumed

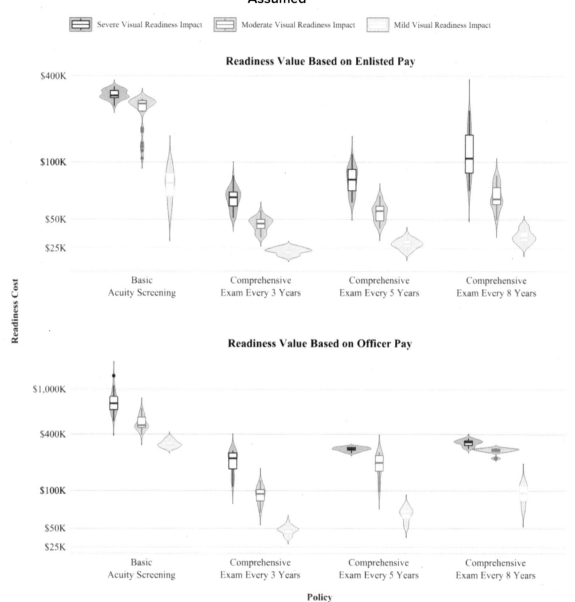

Focusing on the plot depicting the pessimistic case (Figure 3.4), we observe that despite the model's sensitivity to testing specificities, our general finding that comprehensive eye exams significantly reduce readiness costs remains robust. Therefore, this finding can be considered reliable and consistent across different scenarios.

Total Other Costs of Screening Policies

Figure 3.5 presents combined violin and box plots, providing a visual comparison of the distribution of lifetime total other costs across four distinct policy options, various assumptions for the value κ, and separate comparisons for enlisted SM and officer pay trajectories. These total other costs encompass exam costs, treatment costs, potential replacement costs, and discharge costs. In contrast to the earlier readiness costs, which represent benefits from identifying otherwise undiagnosed OVDs, these costs represent the downsides of additional examinations—namely, the exam process itself and the impact on the force of an unsuccessful treatment, resulting in discharging an SM who otherwise would have gone undiagnosed and stayed in service.

Our analysis reveals an interesting finding regarding the comprehensive eye examination policy. The higher costs associated with the comprehensive policy stem from the additional expenses related to the comprehensive eye exams and the inclusion of treatments that may not have been pursued otherwise. This comprehensive policy accounts for the exam costs, treatments, and even the costs incurred by discharging and replacing SMs who may have continued serving had their condition not been detected through the more frequent exams. Moreover, as expected, the significance of κ does not play a role in influencing the total cost outcomes. Instead, the key factor driving the differences in total other costs lies in the increased expense of conducting more frequent comprehensive eye exams. The increase, although statistically significant, ranges between approximately 10 and 15 percent.

Notably, among the policies involving comprehensive eye exams, the frequency of the exams does not have a statistically significant impact on total other costs for enlisted pay trajectories. However, for officer pay, the frequency of exams exhibits a stronger influence on total other costs. This difference arises due to the disparity in discharge costs between officers and enlisted SMs for individuals diagnosed with OVDs that are not effectively treated. Discharge costs for officers are considerably higher and escalate more rapidly with age. Consequently, less frequent comprehensive eye exams for officers elevate the risk of undiagnosed OVDs persisting for extended periods, resulting in officers

36

serving longer before diagnosis and discharge. This prolongation leads to significantly larger discharge costs once officers are discharged prior to their retirement age.

The comprehensive eye exam policy, despite its anticipated benefits, exhibits increased overall costs. Furthermore, the frequency of exams displays varying impacts on total other costs depending on the type of SM, with costs based on officer pay experiencing more pronounced effects due to discharge cost considerations.

Figure 3.5. Total Other Costs per 1,000 Enlisted Service Members of Different Screening or Comprehensive Eye Exam Policies, by Assumed Impact of Undiagnosed Ocular and Visual Dysfunction on Visual Readiness and by Full Readiness Value

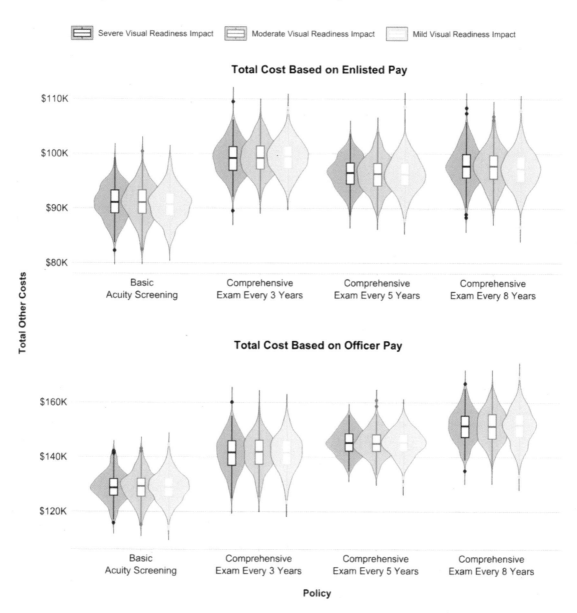

NOTE: Color coding corresponds to the assumed impact of an undiagnosed OVD on visual readiness values. Green corresponds to *mild visual readiness impact* (i.e., where undiagnosed SMs still contribute readiness value, but their contribution is reduced by half); blue to *moderate visual readiness impact* (i.e., where an undiagnosed OVD reduces the visual readiness value contributions of an SM completely to zero); and red to *severe visual readiness impact* (i.e., where an undiagnosed SM subtracts from force readiness by one-half of their fully healthy visual readiness value). The y-axis is total other costs of administering screenings or examinations across the 1,000 simulated SMs and 300 simulated runs, and hence shows total dollar figures for every 1,000 SMs. Box plots indicate the interquartile range (white rectangle) and median (horizontal line in this rectangle), while violin plots show probability density function based on all runs of each policy frequency and readiness value reduction scenario. We vary the value of full visual readiness illustratively based on either average enlisted or officer pay trajectories.

The Net Monetary Benefit

Figure 3.6 displays combined violin and box plots, offering a visual comparison of the distribution of deployable lifetime NMB per SM. The comparison includes three comprehensive eye exam policies relative to the current screening policy, along with various assumptions for the value κ. Additionally, the violin and box plots are presented separately for the enlisted and officer pay trajectories, providing insights specific to these categories. By analyzing the NMB distribution, we can assess the financial benefits associated with the comprehensive eye exam policies compared with current screening. Furthermore, we can evaluate the impact of different assumptions for the value κ on the NMB outcomes.

The distribution of NMB values across all case runs demonstrates a positive correlation between NMB and frequency of exams. This correlation indicates that more frequent comprehensive eye exams are more cost-effective compared with current screenings and to less frequent comprehensive eye exams. Consistent with expectations, the NMB attains its highest value for comprehensive eye exams when the assumed negative impact of readiness of an undiagnosed OVD is severe (i.e., the κ value is negative).

Moreover, we note that there are benefits associated with comprehensive eye examination policies that we do not quantify, and thus do not include in our model. These include improved occupational sorting, records that may improve the sensitivity and specificity of subsequent eye examinations given these exams at accession, and records that establish whether any conditions are preexisting, aiding in subsequent service-connectedness determinations. Although these benefits are not easily incorporated into our model, we would expect them to further increase the benefits of comprehensive eye exams beyond the already positive NMB values shown above.

Tables 3.1 and 3.2 provide comprehensive details regarding the outputs obtained from our CEA. These tables present average NMB values across all case runs for both enlisted and officer pay trajectories, considering various assumptions for the value κ. Additionally, they showcase the differences in average costs and RYG associated with different comprehensive eye exam policies and frequencies compared with the current screening policy. Given that the average NMB values are all positive, it is unsurprising that the RYG values are also positive, indicating a gain in readiness years. Finally, our CEA provides insights into the assumed value per SM year to adopt the corresponding comprehensive policy. As previously described, we calculate λ_{max}, which represents this threshold willingness to pay, by first summing the differences in average costs to obtain our estimate for the expected accrued cost difference as ΔC_F. We then divide this accrued cost difference by the average RYG. This metric helps quantify the monetary value that decisionmakers would consider appropriate for implementing a specific comprehensive eye exam policy.

Figure 3.6. Net Monetary Cost per 1,000 Enlisted Service Members of Different Comprehensive Eye Exam Policies Relative to Current Acuity Screening Policy, by Assumed Impact of Undiagnosed Ocular and Visual Dysfunction on Visual Readiness and by Full Readiness Value

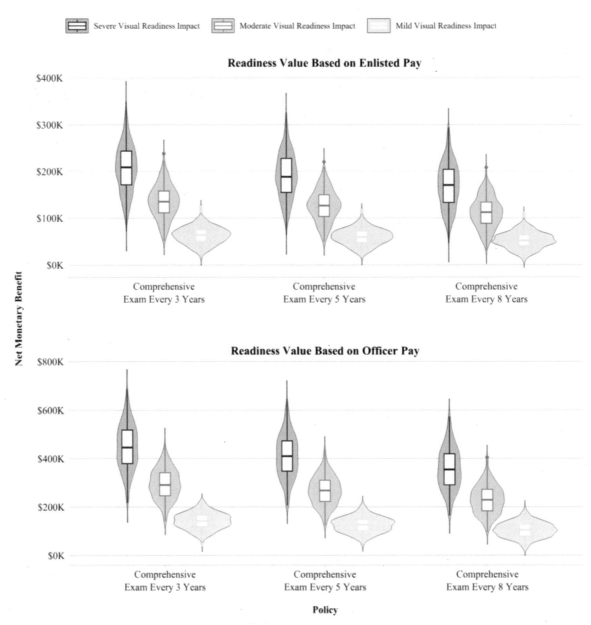

NOTE: Color coding corresponds to the assumed impact of an undiagnosed OVD on visual readiness values. Green corresponds to *mild visual readiness impact* (i.e., where undiagnosed SMs still contribute readiness value, but their contribution is reduced by half); blue to *moderate visual readiness impact* (i.e., where an undiagnosed OVD reduces the visual readiness value contributions of an SM completely to zero); and red to *severe visual readiness impact* (i.e., where an undiagnosed SM subtracts from force readiness by one-half of their fully healthy visual readiness value).The y-axis is the NMB, our measure of cost-effectiveness, resulting from undertaking exam policy under consideration across the 1,000 SMs and 300 simulated runs, and hence shows total dollar figures for every 1,000 SMs. Box plots indicate the interquartile range (white rectangle) and median (horizontal line in this rectangle), while violin plots show probability density function based on all runs of each policy frequency and readiness value reduction scenario. We vary the value of full visual readiness illustratively based on either the average enlisted or officer pay trajectories.

Table 3.1. Cost-Effectiveness Analysis Based on Enlisted Service Member Pay of Comprehensive Eye Exams Relative to Current Basic Acuity Screening Policy

Negative Impact on Readiness of OVD (κ)	Policy and Screening Frequency	Average NMB	Difference in Exam vs. Screening Cost	Difference in Treatment Cost	Difference in Other Costs	Difference in Discharge Cost	RYG	Benefits	Assumed Value per SM Year
Severe	Comprehensive eye exam every three years	$210,000	$500	$1,500	$28,000	-$22,000	2.8	$215,000	$3,000
Severe	Comprehensive eye exam every five years	$190,000	$600	$1,000	$16,000	-$12,500	2.6	$195,000	$2,100
Severe	Comprehensive eye exam every eight years	$170,000	$600	$800	$10,000	-$4,500	2.3	$175,000	$3,000
Moderate	Comprehensive eye exam every three years	$135,000	$500	$1,500	$28,000	-$22,000	1.9	$145,000	$4,400
Moderate	Comprehensive eye exam every five years	$125,000	$600	$1,000	$16,000	-$13,000	1.8	$135,000	$3,000
Moderate	Comprehensive eye exam every eight years	$110,000	$600	$800	$10,000	-$4,800	1.6	$120,000	$4,300
Mild	Comprehensive eye exam every three years	$63,000	$500	$1,500	$28,000	-$21,500	0.9	$71,500	$9,200
Mild	Comprehensive eye exam every five years	$60,000	$600	$1,000	$16,000	-$12,500	0.9	$65,500	$6,600
Mild	Comprehensive eye exam every eight years	$52,000	$600	$700	$10,000	-$4,800	0.8	$58,500	$8,600

Table 3.2. Cost-Effectiveness Analysis Based on Officer Service Member Pay of Comprehensive Eye Exams Relative to Current Basic Acuity Screening Policy

Negative Impact on Readiness of OVD (κ)	Policy and Frequency	NMB	Difference in Exam vs. Screening Cost	Difference in Treatment Cost	Difference in Other Costs	Difference in Discharge Cost	RYG	Benefits	Maximum Willingness to Pay
Severe	Comprehensive eye exam every three years	$755,000	$600	$2,200	$40,500	-$30,000	6	$770,000	$2,100
Severe	Comprehensive eye exam every five years	$695,000	$700	$1,900	$30,500	-$17,000	5.6	$710,000	$3,000
Severe	Comprehensive eye exam every eight years	$610,000	$800	$1,600	$22,000	-$1,900	4.9	$635,000	$4,600
Moderate	Comprehensive eye exam every three years	$505,000	$600	$2,200	$40,500	-$30,500	4	$515,000	$3,200
Moderate	Comprehensive eye exam every five years	$460,000	$700	$1,900	$30,500	-$17,000	3.8	$475,000	$4,400
Moderate	Comprehensive eye exam every eight years	$405,000	$800	$1,600	$22,000	-$2,200	3.3	$425,000	$6,800
Mild	Comprehensive eye exam every three years	$245,000	$600	$2,200	$40,000	-$30,500	2	$260,000	$6,200
Mild	Comprehensive eye exam every five years	$220,000	$700	$1,900	$30,500	-$17,000	1.9	$240,000	$8,800
Mild	Comprehensive eye exam every eight years	$190,000	$800	$1,600	$22,000	-$2,100	1.6	$215,000	$13,500

Varying Readiness Values

In Chapter 2, we presented the visual readiness values associated with enlisted SMs and officers as a function of age in Figure 2.4. These readiness values were estimated based on RMC, which includes monthly pay, housing allowances, and subsistence allowances by pay grade for both enlisted and officer SMs. However, it is important to note that the visual readiness provided by SMs may exceed their compensation and allowances. To explore this further, we investigated how the readiness cost changes for different screening policies when an SM's readiness value is assumed to be 50 percent and 100 percent higher than their compensation and allowances.

Figure 3.7 displays combined violin and box plots, allowing for a separate comparison of the distribution of deployable lifetime readiness costs per SM in the case of zero κ, or the moderate impact of undiagnosed OVD on readiness; we chose zero κ (or moderate visual readiness reduction) to illustrate a case to represent a middle scenario. Negative or positive κ scenarios would vary qualitatively accordingly to the above analysis. This comparison is made across four distinct policies, and assumptions concerning the rate at which readiness value increases with age, specifically for enlisted or officer pay trajectories.

As expected, we observe that as we attribute more visual readiness value to SMs beyond their compensation and allowances, the readiness cost of having SMs with undiagnosed OVDs also increases. Additionally, the difference in visual readiness cost between the comprehensive eye exam policies and the acuity screening policy widens. Unsurprisingly, this suggests that since our comprehensive eye exam policies are deemed cost-effective when readiness is estimated to correspond to an SM's compensation and allowances, they remain cost-effective when readiness is estimated to increase at a higher rate with age than compensation and allowances.

Figure 3.7. Total Readiness Cost per 1,000 Enlisted Service Members of Different Screening or Comprehensive Eye Exam Policies, Assuming Moderate Impact on Readiness and Different Readiness Value Assumptions

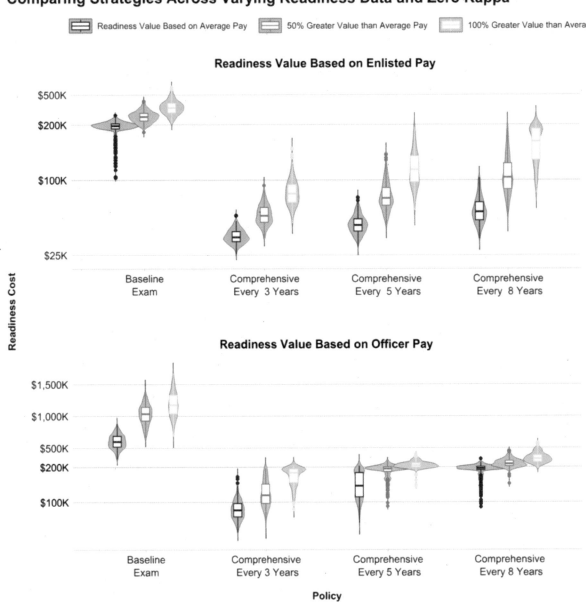

NOTE: All scenarios assume *moderate visual readiness impact* (i.e., where an undiagnosed OVD reduces the visual readiness value contributions of an SM completely to zero). The y-axis is the readiness cost of an undiagnosed OVD, resulting from undertaking exam policy under consideration across the 1,000 SMs and 300 simulated runs, and hence shows total dollar figures for every 1,000 SMs. Box plots indicate the interquartile range (white rectangle) and median (horizontal line in this rectangle), while violin plots show probability density function based on all runs of each policy frequency and readiness value reduction scenario. We vary the value of full visual readiness illustratively based on either average enlisted or officer pay trajectories. Readiness values for fully visually fit SMs are assumed to be the same as in Figure 3.2 (green), 50 percent larger than those values (purple), or 100 percent larger than those values (yellow).

Analysis of the Visual Readiness Trajectories of Service Members for Different Examination Policies

The results presented in our analysis thus far have focused on averages and distributions across the 1,000 case runs of our simulation model. These aggregated results provide a high-level overview of the model's outcomes. It is important to note that these results are derived from averages themselves, as they represent the aggregated values across SMs within each case run and are then averaged across all case runs. Consequently, it is expected that the distributions depicted by our violin plots exhibit a bell-shaped curve, in line with the central limit theorem, which states that averages of random variables tend to follow a Gaussian distribution. However, at the individual level, readiness trajectories of SMs can vary significantly due to stochastic events that average out at the population level.

To gain a deeper understanding of the model's dynamics and the impact of different examination strategies on the distribution of an SM's visual readiness values, we need to examine the results at the SM level. While it is possible to analyze the trajectories of a single SM over time, these trajectories are subject to abrupt changes driven by chance events. Thus, relying on one or a few individual trajectories is insufficient to fully comprehend how visual readiness evolves over time for SMs during service. Instead, we analyze how the distributions of visual readiness for the entire cohort of 300 SMs evolve as they age, specifically by selecting a few representative case runs from our simulation model results. These representative case runs correspond to the median, first quartile, and third quartile of readiness costs across all four screening policies. To illustrate the dynamics of the model, we focus just on the examples of enlisted pay trajectory SMs where κ is assumed to be negative, hence providing the greatest differentiation between fully visually fit SMs and SMs with undiagnosed OVDs.

Figure 3.8 illustratively depicts the dynamics of the readiness distribution using enlisted individual-level trajectories derived from these three representative case runs, focusing on the negative κ case to illustrate most clearly the impact of not regularly screening for undiagnosed OVDs. The plots illustrate how the distribution of visual readiness values evolves over time for each screening policy, starting from $0 and expanding as SMs age. Notably, the current policy acuity screening exhibits a wide distribution of visual readiness values, including individuals who acquire OVDs but remain undiagnosed while still serving. As we transition to comprehensive eye exam policies with increased frequency of scheduled exams, the distribution narrows and progressively aligns with the mean trajectory, representing visual positive readiness. The inclusion of individual trajectories within the distribution provides confidence in the statistical results and offers a more thorough understanding of why comprehensive eye exam policies increase visual readiness values over time—namely, by detecting and treating OVDs earlier.

In this chapter, we implemented the model described in Chapter 2 to estimate the costs, benefits, and net monetary benefits of comprehensive eye exams relative to current basic acuity screening policy. We ran these modeling simulations across a wide range of assumptions and populations, most notably by readiness value based on average enlisted versus officer pay trajectories, by the assumed impact of undiagnosed OVDs on force readiness, and by the assumed accuracy of comprehensive eye exams themselves. As discussed in the Summary, we consistently found that periodic comprehensive eye exams are cost-effective relative to the current policy of basic acuity screenings due to reducing the number of SMs with undiagnosed OVDs, as well as the duration of service of SMs with these undiagnosed OVDs. We turn to a discussion of the limitations of the model and our policy conclusions in Chapter 4.

Figure 3.8. Trajectories of Cumulative Contributions to Visual Readiness by Each Service Member of 1,000 Simulated Service Members, Enlisted Pay, Severe Impact on Readiness Assumption, by Screening or Exam Policy

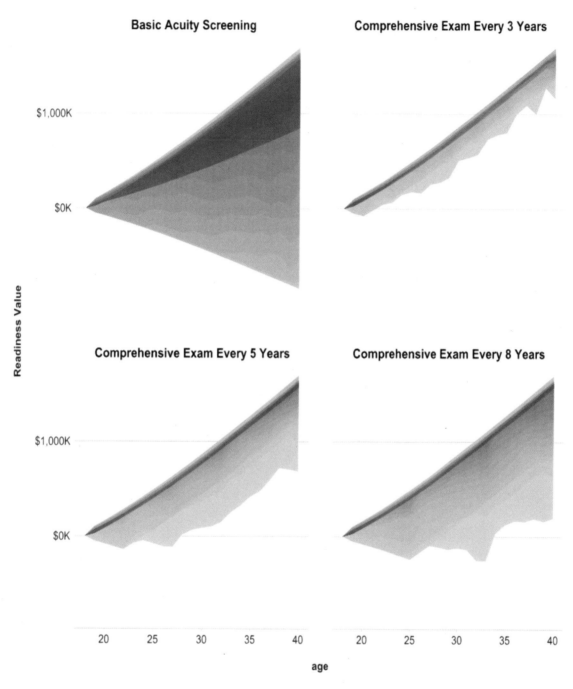

NOTE: The assumed scenario is based on the enlisted pay trajectory and the *severe visual readiness impact* of an undiagnosed OVD. Greater concentrations of SMs are represented by darker colors.

Chapter 4

Limitations, Conclusions, and Recommendations

In this study, we have modeled how the net benefits of comprehensive eye exam policies intend to detect a fuller range of OVDs compare with the current policy of basic acuity screenings. We have found that comprehensive eye exams are cost-effective relative to current policy, and hence we recommend their introduction for a broad range of SMs.

While our research and model exhibit several assumptions and limitations deserving discussion and acknowledgment, not all of them have been explicitly outlined in the description of our model. We discuss them at length in Appendix B, but we note a few prominent assumptions and limitations here before concluding.

In choosing our modeling approach, we prioritized a microsimulation model over simpler and faster-to-run models like expectation or differential equation models. This decision stemmed from the unique demands of our study and the intricate nature of military health care dynamics. While microsimulation models provide the flexibility to capture detailed individual-level interactions, they come with the drawback of being more challenging to comprehend and slower to execute due to their inherent incorporation of chance-driven effects.

A key limitation is that our model lacks extensive external validation of our model output with empirical data. This limitation is not inherent in the model but instead derives from the justification for this analysis to begin with: current screening policy is not designed to systematically detect the prevalence and incidence of a wide array of OVDs among a representative group of SMs, nor of the likely treatment efficacy or impacts on productivity or the force of these OVDs. As such, we recognize that the administration of comprehensive eye exams will allow for much greater certainty; our recommendation of introducing these exams would also allow for more accurately quantifying their costs and benefits for different types of SMs.

But we were able to address this limitation by implementing face validation and sensitivity analysis; these complementary approaches were essential for ensuring the accuracy and reliability of our findings. For face validation, we engaged stakeholders, including eye health specialists from the Vision Center on Excellence, in regular meetings. Through these sessions, we carefully examined the model's assumptions, parameters, and outputs, seeking valuable insights and feedback to align the model with real-world scenarios. This collaborative process bolstered our confidence in the model's representation of complex dynamics within the military setting. Key to our modeling efforts was the understanding that there is not widespread agreement on specific values for important parameters of the model. Therefore, we simultaneously conducted a series sensitivity analysis to assess how changes in various parameters affected the model's behavior and outcomes.

We sought to align examination frequencies with cognitive examinations aimed to streamline the process and ensure consistency in examination protocols. As part of our sensitivity analysis, we introduced an eight-year examination option to explore the model's sensitivity to frequency variations. However, it is essential to recognize that this addition does not eliminate all uncertainties surrounding examination frequencies; further refinement and validation may be necessary to better understand the long-term implications of less frequent exams and their impact on readiness and health care costs.

A primary driver of our results is how we model the benefits of comprehensive eye exams. We do this by assuming that SMs contribute "visual readiness value" to the force while serving—that is, we assume a monetary value of an SM being fully visually fit in order to calculate a benefit from treating otherwise undiagnosed OVDs (thereby restoring the SM to full visual fitness). This use of the word *readiness* does not correspond to existing binary classifications of whether an SM is deployable or retainable, since we assume that absent these comprehensive eye exams, undiagnosed OVDs would continue to go undetected.

Thus, a notable limitation arises in our estimation of visual readiness reduction attributed to undiagnosed OVDs, which hinges on quantifying the influence of these undiagnosed OVDs on SMs' visual readiness. To mitigate reliance on specific assumptions, we varied this impact across a spectrum of values; however, these quantities persist as a fundamental source of uncertainty. Specifically, readiness reduction is contingent on the prevalence and incidence of these OVDs among SMs, particularly with YOS, introducing uncertainty. Consequently, we primarily drew on estimates from the civilian literature and engaged in discussions with DoD SMEs to inform our model.

With these ranges of prevalence and incidence estimates of OVDs, we then turned to quantifying visual readiness and the negative impact of undiagnosed OVDs, which may inadequately capture its multifaceted nature across occupational specialties and pay grades. While assigning a monetary value to optimal visual health for each SM, readiness is heterogeneous and influenced by various factors such as occupation, job-specific skills, and task. Despite deliberately focusing on readiness values based on enlisted or officer pay trajectories to account for various aspects of readiness within the military, this approach may not fully encapsulate the diversity of military roles and responsibilities. Furthermore, linking readiness to pay trajectory, while pragmatic, may oversimplify this multifaceted concept, although we conduct analyses where we further vary these values.

Moreover, our model concentrates on individual-level dynamics of readiness reduction, neglecting to explicitly model broader consequences such as impacts on team composition or unit cohesion. Our assumption of strictly additive OVD impacts implies a consistent marginal effect regardless of the number of affected SMs—that is, that the marginal impact of a new undiagnosed OVD is the same whether there is one SM with an undiagnosed OVD or one hundred. However, this simplification may overlook the ripple effects of replacing SMs with treatment failure on the broader military system, indicating a limitation in the scope of our analysis. Future studies should consider alternative constructions of visual readiness to comprehensively understand this critical aspect of visual fitness. Finally, we assume there is no interaction between the onset of an OVD and other factors that could affect attrition, and thus we assume that "all-other-case" attrition remains unchanged.

But despite these limitations, our model produces the consistently strong conclusion of the cost-effectiveness of comprehensive eye exams that is robust to the uncertainties in parameter values. We note a final limitation that likely increases the cost-effectiveness of comprehensive eye exams: We did not include the full range of potential benefits of comprehensive eye exams at accession and throughout service due to difficulty in quantifying them. These unquantified potential benefits include improved accuracy in establishing service-connectedness of OVDs during the Veterans Affairs disability claims process, improved OVD diagnostic accuracy throughout an SM's career due to improved baseline measures, reduced medical spending due to early detection and successful treatment, and improved sorting into occupational specialty through this comprehensive baseline examination. Adding these benefits would increase the cost-effectiveness of comprehensive eye exams even more than our model suggests, further justifying our recommendation to introduce baseline and periodic comprehensive eye exams for all SMs.

Conclusions and Implications

Despite the increase in total costs of administering periodic comprehensive eye exams to all SMs, our CBA reveals that the reduction in visual readiness costs from early diagnosis outweighed these additional expenses, making the implementation of periodic comprehensive eye exam policy among current SMs cost beneficial. This finding holds even without including the difficult-to-quantify benefits of comprehensive eye exams, such as improved occupational sorting, more thorough medical documentation of visual fitness, and long-term reductions in medical costs or assistive technology expenditures based on early detection and treatment.

Based on these findings, we recommend the introduction of periodic comprehensive eye exams, especially for SMs for whom the negative impacts of undiagnosed OVDs on contributions to the force are high. That is, for occupations for which visual readiness is most pivotal, the cost-effectiveness of comprehensive eye exams is highest. We note that in addition to the benefits quantified above, any systematic expansion of comprehensive eye exams would enable a greater understanding of the prevalence, incidence, and costs of OVDs among the unique SM population, helping future modeling efforts and vision-related policies.

Tables of Numerical Results

This appendix provides tables of the results presented in Chapter 3 that were shown as box and violin plots. We first present tables regarding enlisted SM pay trajectories, showing their readiness cost and total other costs (Tables A.1 and A.2). We then present the same set of tables for officer pay trajectories (Tables A.3 and A.4).

Table A.1. Readiness Cost for Enlisted Service Members

Screening Policy	Mean	Median	1st Quartile	3rd Quartile
Panel A: Readiness cost for enlisted SMs and severe readiness impact of OVDs.				
Baseline visual acuity screening	$280,000	$283,900	$239,800	$315,500
Comprehensive eye exam every three years	$70,000	$65,000	$58,200	$71,900
Comprehensive eye exam every five years	$80,000	$83,100	$73,000	$92,500
Comprehensive eye exam every eight years	$100,000	$102,400	$90,100	$115,700
Panel B: Readiness cost for enlisted SMs and moderate readiness impact of OVDs				
Baseline visual acuity screening	$190,000	$189,100	$162,500	$212,600
Comprehensive eye exam every three years	$40,000	$42,800	$38,500	$48,400
Comprehensive eye exam every five years	$60,000	$54,700	$48,700	$60,900
Comprehensive eye exam every eight years	$70,000	$67,900	$59,400	$77,400
Panel C: Readiness cost for enlisted SMs and mild readiness impact of OVDs.				
Baseline visual acuity screening	$90,000	$94,500	$81,200	$105,600
Comprehensive eye exam every three years	$20,000	$21,600	$19,500	$23,900
Comprehensive eye exam every five years	$30,000	$27,700	$24,400	$30,400
Comprehensive eye exam every eight years	$30,000	$34,000	$29,800	$38,600

Table A.2. Total Other Costs for Enlisted Service Members

Screening Policy	Mean	Median	1st Quartile	3rd Quartile
Panel A: Total other costs for enlisted SMs and severe readiness impact of OVDs.				
Baseline visual acuity screening	$90,000	$91,100	$89,100	$93,300
Comprehensive eye exam every three years	$100,000	$99,200	$96,900	$101,300
Comprehensive eye exam every five years	$100,000	$96,500	$94,500	$98,300
Comprehensive eye exam every eight years	$100,000	$97,800	$95,700	$99,900
Panel B: Total other costs for enlisted SMs and moderate readiness impact of OVDs.				
Baseline visual acuity screening	$90,000	$91,100	$89,000	$93,300
Comprehensive eye exam every three years	$100,000	$99,200	$97,200	$101,400
Comprehensive eye exam every five years	$100,000	$96,300	$94,100	$98,300
Comprehensive eye exam every eight years	$100,000	$97,800	$95,500	$99,700
Panel C: Total other costs for enlisted SMs and mild readiness impact of OVDs.				
Baseline visual acuity screening	$90,000	$90,800	$88,600	$92,800
Comprehensive eye exam every three years	$100,000	$99,500	$97,300	$101,400
Comprehensive eye exam every five years	$100,000	$96,200	$94,300	$98,300
Comprehensive eye exam every eight years	$100,000	$97,300	$94,900	$99,500

Table A.3. Readiness Cost for Officers

Screening Policy	Mean	Median	1st Quartile	3rd Quartile
Panel A: Readiness cost for officers and severe readiness impact of OVDs.				
Baseline visual acuity screening	$900,000	$905,900	$790,800	$1,028,400
Comprehensive eye exam every three years	$130,000	$130,200	$114,800	$147,500
Comprehensive eye exam every five years	$190,000	$187,700	$162,000	$217,700
Comprehensive eye exam every eight years	$270,000	$261,800	$225,800	$306,100
Panel B: Readiness cost for officers and moderate readiness impact of OVDs.				
Baseline visual acuity screening	$600,000	$599,200	$520,700	$686,700

Screening Policy	Mean	Median	1st Quartile	3rd Quartile
Comprehensive eye exam every three years	$90,000	$87,400	$77,200	$98,100
Comprehensive eye exam every five years	$130,000	$125,400	$108,000	$145,900
Comprehensive eye exam every eight years	$180,000	$177,500	$150,800	$204,500
Panel C: Readiness cost for officers and mild readiness impact of OVDs.				
Baseline visual acuity screening	$300,000	$304,800	$262,100	$344,000
Comprehensive eye exam every three years	$40,000	$43,700	$39,000	$48,900
Comprehensive eye exam every five years	$60,000	$63,700	$54,300	$72,800
Comprehensive eye exam every eight years	$90,000	$87,900	$75,100	$102,800

Table A.4. Total Other Costs for Officers

Screening Policy	Mean	Median	1st Quartile	3rd Quartile
Panel A: Total other costs for officers and severe readiness impact of OVDs.				
Baseline visual acuity screening	$130,000	$128,600	$125,800	$131,900
Comprehensive eye exam every three years	$140,000	$141,700	$137,000	$145,900
Comprehensive eye exam every five years	$150,000	$145,200	$142,200	$148,600
Comprehensive eye exam every eight years	$150,000	$151,400	$147,400	$155,200
Panel B: Total other costs for officers and moderate readiness impact of OVDs.				
Baseline visual acuity screening	$130,000	$129,200	$125,500	$132,100
Comprehensive eye exam every three years	$140,000	$141,900	$137,300	$146,100
Comprehensive eye exam every five years	$150,000	$144,900	$142,200	$148,200
Comprehensive eye exam every eight years	$150,000	$151,300	$146,800	$155,800
Panel C: Total other costs for officers and mild readiness impact of OVDs.				
Baseline visual acuity screening	$130,000	$128,800	$125,500	$132,200
Comprehensive eye exam every three years	$140,000	$141,600	$137,300	$146,000
Comprehensive eye exam every five years	$150,000	$145,300	$142,300	$148,400
Comprehensive eye exam every eight years	$150,000	$151,800	$147,500	$155,800

Sensitivity Analysis and Modeling Limitations

In our sensitivity analysis, we aimed to determine the leverage of each input variable on the model outputs, particularly focusing on the readiness value. The leverage of an input variable refers to how sensitive the output values are to changes in that specific input variable. To quantify this relationship and gain insights into the importance of different inputs on the outputs, we calculated Spearman's PRCC between the model input parameters and the outputs.

The PRCC measures the degree of association between a model output and a model input while controlling for the effects of other inputs. By considering the influence of confounding variables, it enhances the accuracy of assessing the relationship between inputs and outputs. Through the use of the PRCC, we gain a deeper understanding of the relationships between inputs and outputs in our simulation model. This understanding enables us to identify critical factors that significantly affect the model's behavior and outcomes. By identifying and evaluating these influential factors, we can make informed decisions and recommendations regarding policies and their potential effects on the model outputs.

The plots presented in Figures B.1 and B.2 provide a visual representation of the PRCCs between the model inputs and readiness outcomes. This plot allows us to analyze the influence of various

Figure B.1. Partial Rank Correlation Coefficients from Sensitivity Analysis Based on Uniform Sampling Distribution

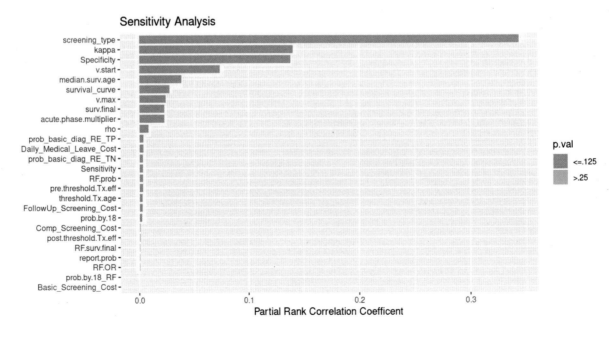

parameters on the overall readiness. The first plot (Figure B.1) is with sampling specificity using a uniform distribution, and the second (Figure B.2) is with sampling specificity using a PERT distribution (a subset of the beta class of distributions), where the greatest weight is placed on larger specificities; they both follow the same format as that described in Chapter 3.

Figure B.2. Partial Rank Correlation Coefficients from Sensitivity Analysis Based on PERT Sampling Distribution

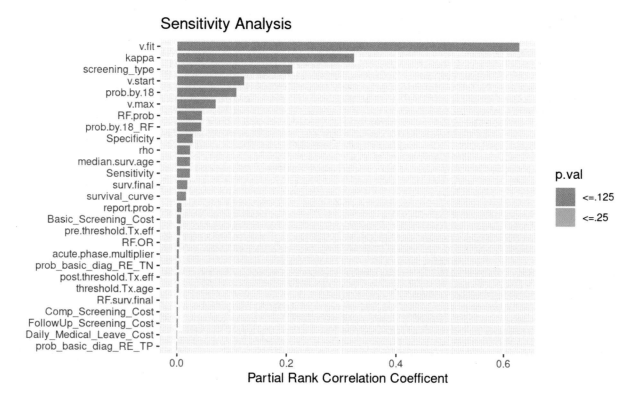

Modeling Limitations

We recognize that our model has several limitations, many of which stem from strategic simplifications made to balance model parsimony and accuracy. To ensure robust results within the uncertainty ranges of model parameter values, we conducted sensitivity analysis and designed experiments to consider a wide range of possible outcomes. Despite these efforts, it is important to acknowledge some key limitations of our model, which we outline below.

Informing the Model

The model considers seven OVDs and includes many parameters whose range of values must be estimated. Many of these parameters have large uncertainties. For example, estimating the value of SMs that have undiagnosed OVDs and therefore reduced vision fitness relative to SMs without OVDs presents challenges based on the potential severity of each OVD and the duty requirements of each SM. By exploring a large number of model outcomes using unique combinations of plausible parameter values in the model, we can identify which policies consistently outperform others while being robust to the underlying uncertainties in parameter value estimates.

Data Limitations

A notable limitation of our analysis is the reliance on estimating incidence curves for OVDs solely based on existing literature. Unfortunately, we lacked access to individual-level or aggregated-level military data based on comprehensive eye exams of a representative set of SMs, which could have informed more accurate incidence curves for different OVDs based on incidence and prevalence rates within military populations across various age groups. To address this data gap, we conducted uncertainty analysis, considering a wide range of values to specify the survival curves. While this approach helped to account for the lack of data, we note that even if we had access to military data, these data would not be representative of all SMs, and thus we would have had to conduct similar analysis and our results would likely be unchanged. Because there are not systematic, regular comprehensive eye exams administered for the military population currently, the existing data on incidence and prevalence are likely biased, since comprehensive eye exams currently need to be "triggered" by another health condition or be directly indicated due to severity.

Sources of Modeling Heterogeneity

The model does not consider many significant demographic and occupational differences in costs and benefits from comprehensive eye examinations. Currently, it only considers age and how various risks associated with developing OVDs change with age. Additionally, treatment and readiness costs are assumed to apply equally to all SMs considered in the model. Significant heterogeneities include gender, military occupational specialty, rank, and deployment status. Adding additional heterogeneity requires informing the model with regression-based models that estimate how costs and risks change with these other attributes, although the model can be run with different parameter estimates that reflect costs and benefits for different groups of SMs.

Indeed, the different assumptions over the impact of OVDs on visual readiness value, as well as the visual readiness value of a given SM, can be interpreted as different types of SMs with particularly high readiness value or for whom visual fitness is most important for fulfilling duties.

We use a common assumption over incidence of TBI and OVDs; alternative risks could be factored into our model to quantify the frequency and the level of environmental severity that SMs are exposed to when deployed. However, we are unaware of data we can use to accurately quantify increased hazard rates for the OVDs we consider, and resulting increases in likelihood of OVDs, during these periods of increased environmental exposure.

Incidence Models

As described in the section "Survival or Nonincidence Models" in Chapter 2, we assume two simple models that determine the yearly probability of developing an RF or an OVD. The simplest of the two assumes an exponential *survival*, or incidence, model, translating to a constant annual probability associated with these risks. For example, we assume that the RF for VDTBI is whether or not an SM has ever had a TBI, and we assume that the yearly probability of having a TBI is constant, although we have explored other assumptions with limited impact on our overall findings.

Attrition and Other Health Factors

The model focuses on SM attrition caused by being diagnosed with an OVD that can no longer be treated, assuming an all-other-cause attrition rate to factor in background attrition effects unrelated to SMs' visual fitness. However, our model does not explicitly describe each type of SM attrition. Instead, it groups all these types into a single all-other-cause rate, which is assumed to be independent of undiagnosed OVDs. If undiagnosed OVDs are correlated with other health conditions or reasons for discharge, our findings would thus be biased.

Correlation of Ocular and Visual Dysfunctions

As we have noted, our model assumes that the seven OVDs we model are independent and not causally related or correlated. In our model, the probability that an SM develops an OVD does not change and depends on having a different OVD. We have chosen the set of OVDs that best conform to this assumption. For example, VDTBI groups together a set of highly correlated OVDs that depend on having had a TBI; the other six OVDs do not depend on having had a TBI. This assumption can be relaxed. For example, we could specify that an OVD represents an RF of a different OVD, increasing its probability of being acquired.

If the assumption of independence is inaccurate, our model will overestimate the total prevalence of having any OVDs. Hence, in this case our model provides a pessimistic scenario of visual fitness outcomes.

Population-Level Linearity in the Readiness Value

In the simulation model, we make an important assumption regarding the estimation of population-level visual readiness value. We assume that this value can be determined by simply summing up the visual readiness value of each individual SM within the population. This assumption is based on the understanding that in realistic scenarios, the majority of SMs maintain vision fitness throughout their deployable YOS.

However, it is important to acknowledge that this simplifying assumption may become less valid if the rates of acquiring OVDs are significantly higher than our parameter inputs. In such cases, a considerable proportion of SMs may lose visual fitness before reaching the age of 40. To illustrate this, let us consider an example. The marginal impact on readiness of adding one SM with vision fitness will be greater if only 50 percent of a unit is fully visually fit compared with a scenario where 90 percent of the unit is fully visually fit. Therefore, although the linearly additive assumption is generally reasonable, its validity may be compromised when a significant number of SMs experience OVDs during their service, highlighting the need for a more nuanced approach in such cases.

False Positivity Rates and Exams at Accession

Although our comprehensive eye examination scenarios include an eye exam at accession, we did not assume comprehensive eye exams as a determinative entry-level criterion for recruits in our analysis—that is, comprehensive eye exams do not prevent a given recruit from accessing. However, we did consider this hypothetical scenario to understand how using a comprehensive eye exam at entry could affect readiness if the exam were to prevent accession. Our findings reveal that implementing a comprehensive eye exam at entry, which evaluates various OVDs independently, results in a relatively low combined specificity. This low specificity raises the risk of false positive outcomes where individuals without OVDs may be mistakenly identified as having them and thus not access even though they are visually fit.

In contrast, current screening policy, which focuses solely on RE at entry, lowers the likelihood of false positives. Therefore, our simulation model exclusively relies on the baseline screenings of RE as an entry criteria.

We provide detailed findings on the expected false positivity rates for comprehensive eye examinations on entry in Table B.1. The table showcases the average false positive rates for the baseline visual acuity screening at entry and the comprehensive eye exam at entry, as well as the average readiness values for recruited SMs with assumed enlisted pay trajectories throughout their deployable careers.

Table B.1. False Positive Rates and Average Readiness with Replacement

False Positive Rate	Average Readiness Per SM	SM	Strategy
22%	$1,451,815	Enlisted pay	Acuity Screening
40%	$1,637,850	Enlisted pay	Comprehensive eye exam every three years
	$1,623,351	Enlisted pay	Comprehensive eye exam every five years
	$1,610,115	Enlisted pay	Comprehensive eye exam every eight years
22%	$2,238,253	Officer pay	Acuity screening
40%	$2,852,361	Officer pay	Comprehensive eye exam every three years
	$2,808,890	Officer pay	Comprehensive eye exam every five years
	$2,761,617	Officer pay	Comprehensive eye exam every eight years

For the acuity screening at entry, the average false positive rate across our simulated cases is 22 percent. The average visual readiness value for enlisted SMs throughout their service under the acuity screening policy amounts to $1,451,815. Although there is a loss of readiness associated with the low specificity and high false positive rate of the basic acuity screening, it is comparatively smaller than that of the comprehensive eye exam.

For the comprehensive eye exam at entry, the average false positive rate across our simulated cases is 40 percent. The average visual readiness value for enlisted SMs throughout their service under the policy of comprehensive eye exams every three years is $1,637,850. This results in a larger loss of readiness due to the low specificity and high false positive rate associated with the comprehensive eye exam. Results are similar for officers and enlisted pay trajectories.

Appendix C

Estimation of Productivity Loss Associated with Onset of Low Vision in the Adult Civilian Population

In our review of the literature estimating the burden of OVDs on military SMs, we found that the prominent 2019 study by Frick and Singman relied on estimates of the productivity loss associated with OVDs based on 1997 data on adults over the age of 40, using direct comparisons of labor force outcomes between those reporting low vision or blindness and those not reporting these conditions.[1] Although Rein and colleagues used a range of estimates for productivity losses given fundamental uncertainty of this impact in the military context, we undertook a brief analysis to provide an updated estimate to inform future studies relying on estimates of productivity loss associated with OVDs. To do so, we drew on the 2014 and 2018 panels of the Survey of Income and Program Participation (SIPP), a U.S. Census–administered nationally representative survey of households in the United States that follows these households over the course of four years. Each survey year references characteristics from the previous year, so the reference years that our analysis includes span 2013–2020. Rein and colleagues used the 1997 reference year from the 1996 SIPP panel,[2] although we note that the SIPP underwent a substantial redesign with the introduction of the 2014 panel, and hence variables and reference periods are not directly comparable between the 2014 and 1996 SIPP panels.

The SIPP elicits a substantial amount of information about each household member, including sociodemographic characteristics, work activities, economic status, and health status. Most relevantly, interviewers seek an answer to the following question: "Is [the respondent] blind or does he/she have serious difficulty seeing?" Information on other disabilities, functional limitations, and work-limiting health conditions are elicited. Additionally, respondents are asked about their annual earnings and about annual hours worked. Households are reinterviewed annually for up to four years in the panel.

Our event study research design is intended to produce an answer to the question, If a working adult with no work-limiting health conditions begins to have difficulty seeing, how is their work status affected? Intuitively, we answer this question by limiting our sample to respondents who start in the panel working and report no work-limiting health conditions but who report low vision/blindness (answering yes to the above question on being blind or having serious difficulty seeing) *in a subsequent survey*. We then track how their hours worked and earnings differed before and after the onset of a new visual impairment.

---

[1] Frick and Singman, 2019; Rein, Zhang, Wirth, Lee, Hoerger, McCall, Klein, Tielsch, Vijan, and Saaddine, 2006.

[2] Rein, Zhang, Wirth, Lee, Hoerger, McCall, Klein, Tielsch, Vijan, and Saaddine, 2006.

This design is intended to address a major concern with Rein and colleagues' approach comparing work status among individuals reporting low vision with those without low vision.[3] The concern is that this comparison includes both the difference in work status due to low vision and any other factors that differ between these two populations. The SIPP has rich data that allow for many controls (although Rein and colleagues appear to have conducted comparisons without controls),[4] but latent unobserved factors are likely to confound any inference of the productivity losses associated with OVDs. For example, rates of low vision are higher among individuals with diabetes. Diabetes is not directly observed in the SIPP, and thus comparisons in work status across individuals with low vision would conflate the productivity loss we seek to estimate with the productivity loss associated with diabetes. Similar unobserved characteristics could include prior concussions, access to affordable optometric services, access to affordable treatment for visual or ocular disorders, or family history of blindness, among others.

Even if all such factors were controlled for, we argue that the corresponding estimate would be inapplicable to the context at hand. Such an estimate would include congenital or long-running low vision or blindness issues and corresponding life choices (e.g., occupational sorting) resulting in differences in work status. In our context of military SMs who acquire OVDs during service, we instead want to estimate the impact of low vision on readiness. This estimate corresponds to a worker *developing* low vision.

By comparing within-worker changes at the onset of low vision, we both purge our estimate of unobserved differences and focus on the productivity losses associated with loss of vision. We therefore estimate equations of the form

$$(Y_{i,t} - Y_{i,VL-1}) = \alpha + \beta VL_{i,t} + \Gamma X_{i,t} + \epsilon_{i,t}.$$

The indicator VL is one if the individual reports having low vision in year t and zero otherwise. The dependent variable is the change in annual hours worked or annual earnings, comparing year t to the year before first reporting low vision. We condition our sample on those who are working in the first interview year and who do not report low vision or any other disability in that year, so if the onset of low vision occurs in the second interview, then the "baseline" year is the first interview year. The coefficient of interest is β, which is the effect of the indicator variable visual loss (VL) turning from zero to 1. We control for a range of individual characteristics, including race/ethnicity, sex, age, educational attainment, marital status, and rurality, as well as fixed effects for calendar year and state of residence. Robust standard errors are clustered at the individual level, and all regressions are weighted using respondent replicate weights. We include all adults who report working; although we would prefer to limit the sample to those ages 18 to 39, there are too few occurrences of onset of low vision with this restriction to provide sufficient statistical power for inference.

We employed a range of specifications and robustness checks, with two consistent findings: there appeared to be no statistically significant effect of onset of low vision on earnings, and a consistently negative statistically significant effect of between 70 and 140 fewer hours worked per year. Our preferred specification yields an estimate of a statistically significant reduction of 106 hours worked per year in the year of low vision onset. Given average hours worked of 1,824 at baseline, this effect amounts to a 6-percent decrease in hours worked.

---

[3] Rein, Zhang, Wirth, Lee, Hoerger, McCall, Klein, Tielsch, Vijan, and Saaddine, 2006.

[4] Rein, Zhang, Wirth, Lee, Hoerger, McCall, Klein, Tielsch, Vijan, and Saaddine, 2006.

Input Tables

We reviewed 66 articles to obtain the estimates of input parameters for the prevalence of eye conditions. We then calculated the minimum and maximum of distribution of estimates extracted from the literature to inform the model, shown in Table D.1. The lower bounds of RE, glaucoma, and VDTBI, and the upper bounds of RE and glaucoma, have been modified based on the SMEs' opinions. As noted in Table 2.3, the revised estimate for RE is 0.15. We then used these age 18 prevalence numbers and incidence rates to calculate probabilities of not developing visual impairments by age 40.

Table D.1. Prevalence of Condition by Age

Condition/OVD	Fraction of OVD at Age 18	
	Lower	Upper
Corneal dystrophy	0.0009	0.0013[b]
Keratoconus	0.0012[c]	0.009[d]
Retinal dystrophy	0.000033	0.00138[f]
Dry eye	0.002[g]	0.0574[g,h]
Glaucoma	0.0069[h]	0.0789[h]
RE	0.01[i]	0.5[i]
VDTBI	0.02[j]	0.17[j]
VDTBI w/RF	0.23[k]	0.66[l]

[a] J.-L. Bourges, "Corneal Dystrophies," *Journal français d'ophtalmologie*, Vol. 40, No. 6, June 2017.

[b] Musch, D. C., L. M. Niziol, J. D. Stein, R. M. Kamyar, and A. Sugar, "Prevalence of Corneal Dystrophies in the United States: Estimates from Claims Data," *Investigative Ophthalmology and Visual Science*, Vol. 52, No. 9, September 1, 2011.

[c] J. A. P. Gomes, P. F. Rodrigues, and L. L. Lamazales, "Keratoconus Epidemiology: A Review," *Saudi Journal of Ophthalmology*, Vol. 36, No. 1, July 11, 2022.

[d] S. Z. Munir, W. M. Munir, and J. Albrecht, "Estimated Prevalence of Keratoconus in the United States from a Large Vision Insurance Database," *Eye and Contact Lens: Science and Clinical Practice*, Vol. 47, No. 9, September 2021.

[e] H. Chawla and V. Vohra, "Retinal Dystrophies," StatPearls, last updated March 16, 2023.

[f] J. Gong, S. Cheung, A. Fasso-Opie, O. Galvin, L. S. Moniz, D. Earle, T. Durham, J. Menzo, N. Li, S. Duffy, J. Dolgin, et al., "The Impact of Inherited Retinal Diseases in the United States of America (US) and Canada from a Cost-of-Illness Perspective," *Clinical Ophthalmology*, Vol. 15, July 1, 2021.

[g] R. Dandona, L. Dandona, T. J. Naduvilath, M. Srinivas, C. A. McCarty, and G. N. Rao, "Refractive Errors in an Urban Population in Southern India: The Andhra Pradesh Eye Disease Study," *Investigative Ophthalmology and Visual Science*, Vol. 40, No. 12, November 1999.

[h] National Eye Institute, "Glaucoma Tables," last updated February 7, 2020.

[i] S. Vitale, L. Ellwein, M. F. Cotch, F. L. Ferris III, and R. Sperduto, "Prevalence of Refractive Error in the United States, 1999–2004," *Archives of Ophthalmology*, Vol. 126, No. 8, August 2008.

[j] L. H. Trieu and J. B. Lavrich, "Current Concepts in Convergence Insufficiency," *Current Opinion in Ophthalmology*, Vol. 29, No. 5, September 2018.

[k] T. L. Alvarez, E. H. Kim, V. R. Vicci, S. K. Dhar, B. B. Biswal, and A. M. Barrett, "Concurrent Vision Dysfunctions in Convergence Insufficiency with Traumatic Brain Injury," *Optometry and Vision Science*, Vol. 89, No. 12, December 2012.

[l] G. L. Goodrich, H. M. Flyg, J. E. Kirby, C. Y. Chang, and G. L. Martinsen, "Mechanisms of TBI and Visual Consequences in Military and Veteran Populations," *Optometry and Vision Science*, Vol. 90, No. 2, February 2013.

We reviewed 25 articles to find estimates for the input parameter *treatment efficacy*. We then calculated the upper and lower bounds of the distribution of estimates we extracted from the literature, shown in Table D.2 below. As described in the body of the report, we transformed these numbers to calculate the treatment's annual efficacy.

Table D.2. Treatment Efficacy by Condition

Condition/OVD	Treatment End Efficacy as Fraction of Treated OVDs	
Corneal dystrophy	0.14[a]	1[b]
Dry eye	0.21[c]	0.9[d]
Glaucoma	0.35[e]	0.93[f]
Keratoconus	0.02[g]	0.9[h]
RE	0.39[i]	1[j]
Retinal dystrophy	0.31[k]	0.71[l]
VDTBI	0.04[m]	0.92[m]

[a] M. S. Sridhar, C. J. Rapuano, C. B. Cosar, E. J. Cohen, and P. R. Laibson, "Phototherapeutic Keratectomy Versus Diamond Burr Polishing of Bowman's Membrane in the Treatment of Recurrent Corneal Erosions Associated with Anterior Basement Membrane Dystrophy," *Ophthalmology*, Vol. 109, No. 4, April 2002

[b] F. Arnalich-Montiel, J. L. Hernández-Verdejo, N. Oblanca, F. J. Muñoz-Negrete, and M. P. De Miguel, "Comparison of Corneal Haze and Visual Outcome in Primary DSAEK Versus DSAEK Following Failed DMEK," *Graefe's Archive for Clinical and Experimental Ophthalmology*, Vol. 251, No. 11, November 2013.

[c] J. C. Pinto-Bonilla, A. del Olmo-Jimeno, F. Llovet-Osuna, and E. Hernández-Galilea, "A Randomized Crossover Study Comparing Trehalose/Hyaluronate Eyedrops and Standard Treatment: Patient Satisfaction in the Treatment of Dry Eye Syndrome," *Therapeutics and Clinical Risk Management*, Vol. 11, April 13, 2015.

[d] R. M. Shtein, J. F. Shen, A. N. Kuo, K. M. Hammersmith, J. Y. Li, and M. P. Weikert, "Autologous Serum-Based Eye Drops for Treatment of Ocular Surface Disease: A Report by the American Academy of Ophthalmology," *Ophthalmology*, Vol. 127, No. 1, January 2020.

[e] N. D. Baker, H. S. Barnebey, M. R. Moster, M. C. Stiles, S. D. Vold, A. K. Khatana, B. E. Flowers, D. S. Grover, N. G. Strouthidis, J. F. Panarelli/INN005 Study Group, "Ab-Externo MicroShunt Versus Trabeculectomy in Primary Open-Angle Glaucoma: One-Year Results from a 2-Year Randomized, Multicenter Study," *Ophthalmology*, Vol. 128, No. 12, December 2021.

[f] M. A. El Afrit, D. Saadouli, G. Hachicha, K. Ben Mansour, N. El Afrit, and S. Yahyaoui, "The Outcome of Surgical Treatment in Advanced Glaucoma," *Archivos de la Sociedad Española de Oftalmología*, English ed., Vol. 96, No. 4, April 2021.

[g] S. Belviranli and R. Oltulu, "Efficacy of Pulsed-Light Accelerated Crosslinking in the Treatment of Progressive Keratoconus: Two-Year Results," *European Journal of Ophthalmology*, Vol. 30, No. 6, November 2020.

[h] A. Fadlallah, A. Dirani, H. El Rami, G. Cherfane, and E. Jarade, "Safety and Visual Outcome of Visian Toric ICL Implantation After Corneal Collagen Cross-Linking in Keratoconus," *Journal of Refractive Surgery*, Vol. 29, No. 2, February 2013.

[i] J. J. Walline, "Myopia Control: A Review," *Eye and Contact Lens*, Vol. 41, No. 1, January 2016.

[j] C. K. Yim, A. Dave, A. Strawn, J. Chan, I. Zhou, and D. C. Zhu, "Visual Outcomes and Patient Satisfaction After Bilateral Refractive Lens Exchange with a Trifocal Intraocular Lens in Patients with Presbyopia," *Ophthalmology and Therapy*, Vol. 12, No. 3, June 2023.

[k] Y. Rotenstreich, D. Harats, A. Shaish, E. Pras, and M. Belkin, "Treatment of a Retinal Dystrophy, Fundus albipunctatus, with Oral 9-cis-{beta}-Carotene. *British Journal of Ophthalmology*, Vol. 94, No. 5, May 2010.

[l] A. M. Maguire, S. Russell, D. C. Chung, Z. F. Yu, A. Tillman, A. V. Drack, F. Simonelli, B. P. Leroy, K. Z. Reape, K. A. High, et al., "Durability of Voretigene Neparvovec for Biallelic RPE65-Mediated Inherited Retinal Disease: Phase 3 Results at 3 and 4 Years," *Ophthalmology*, Vol. 128, No. 10, October 2021.

[m] J. Johansson, C. Nygren de Boussard, G. Öqvist Seimyr, and T. Pansell, "The Effect of Spectacle Treatment in Patients with Mild Traumatic Brain Injury: A Pilot Study," *Clinical and Experimental Optometry*, Vol. 100, No. 3, May 2017.

We obtained the estimated treatment costs from various online resources cited below. When sources provide the range of estimated costs, we picked the median. We then processed estimates obtained from the literature in two steps to get the minimum and maximum of the distribution, as shown in Table D.3. First, we noted that the estimated costs would cover eye treatments over ten years. Therefore, we divided this number by 10 to get the yearly treatment cost illustrated in the table below. Second, we modified some of the numbers based on SME opinions. For example, the lower bound of VDTBI treatment cost has been reduced to 250, and the upper bound of dry eye treatment cost was increased to 200.

Table D.3. Annual Treatment Costs by Condition

Condition/OVD	Yearly Treatment Cost	
	Lower	Upper
Corneal dystrophy	$1,764.50[a]	$1,988[b]
Dry eye	$78.30[c]	$78.30[c]
Glaucoma	$640	$930[d]
Keratoconus	$115[e]	$2,150[e]
RE	$50[f]	$263.20[g]
Retinal dystrophy	$725[h]	$425,000[i]
VDTBI	$757.20[j]	$757.20[j]

[a] D. K. Dhaliwal, V. Chirikov, J. Schmier, S. Rege, and S. Newton, "Cost Burden of Endothelial Keratoplasty in Fuchs Endothelial Dystrophy: Real-World Analysis of a Commercially Insured US Population (2014–2019)," *Clinical Ophthalmology*, Vol. 16, April 6, 2022.

[b] A. H. Howell, "What's the Average Cost of a Cornea Transplant?" GoodRx, May 11, 2022.

[c] J. Yu, C. V. Asche, and C. J. Fairchild, "The Economic Burden of Dry Eye Disease in the United States: A Decision Tree Analysis," *Cornea*, Vol. 30, No. 4, April 2011.

[d] S. Paretts, "Glaucoma Surgery Cost and Financing," CareCredit, November 3, 2022.

[e] Amplify EyeCare, "How Much Does Keratoconus Treatment Cost?" undated.

[f] CVS, "How Much Do Contacts Cost?" undated.

[g] L. Groth, B. DeBroff, "How Much Does LASIK Eye Surgery Cost in 2024?" *Forbes Health*, 2024.

[h] R. S. Nirwan, T. A. Albini, J. Sridhar, H. W. Flynn Jr., and A. E. Kuriyan, "Assessing 'Cell Therapy' Clinics Offering Treatments of Ocular Conditions Using Direct-to-Consumer Marketing Websites in the United States," *Ophthamology*, Vol. 126, No. 10, October 2019.

[i] S. Scutti, "Gene Therapy for Rare Retinal Disorder to Cost $425,000 per Eye," CNN, January 2, 2018.

[j] Frick and Singman, 2019.

Table D.4. Accuracy of Comprehensive Eye Screening

Condition/OVD	Sensitivity		Specificity	
	Lower	Upper	Lower	Upper
Corneal dystrophy	0.63[a]	0.94[b]	0.73[b]	0.97[b]
Dry eye	0.63[c]	0.98[d]	0.4[d]	1[e]
Keratoconus	0.68[f]	1[g]	0.68[h]	0.9987[i]
RE	0.38[j]	0.978[k]	0.58[l]	0.988[m]
Retinal dystrophy	0.824[n]	1[o]	0.67[p]	0.996[o]
VDTBI	0.78[q]	0.89[q]	0.95[q]	0.98[q]
Glaucoma	0.74[r]	0.93[s]	0.574[s]	0.86[r]

[a] F. Arnalich-Montiel, D. Mingo-Botín, and P. de Arriba-Palomero, "Preoperative Risk Assessment for Progression to Descemet Membrane Endothelial Keratoplasty Following Cataract Surgery in Fuchs Endothelial Corneal Dystrophy," *American Journal of Ophthalmology*, Vol. 208, December 2019.

[b] T. Eleiwa, A. Elsawy, M. Tolba, W. Feuer, S. Yoo, and M. A. Shousha, "Diagnostic Performance of 3-Dimensional Thickness of the Endothelium-Descemet Complex in Fuchs' Endothelial Cell Corneal Dystrophy," *Ophthalmology*, Vol. 127, No. 7, July 2020.

[c] H. B. Hwang, Y. H. Ku, E. C. Kim, H. S. Kim, M. S. Kim, and H. S. Hwang, "Easy and Effective Test to Evaluate Tear-Film Stability for Self-Diagnosis of Dry Eye Syndrome: Blinking Tolerance Time (BTT)," *BMC Ophthalmology*, Vol. 20, No. 1, November 2020.

[d] N. L. Oden, D. E. Lilienfeld, M. A. Lemp, J. D. Nelson, and F. Ederer, "Sensitivity and Specificity of a Screening Questionnaire for Dry Eye," *Advances in Experimental Medicine and Biology*, Vol. 438, 1998.

[e] R Latkany, B. G. Lock, and M. Speaker, "Tear Film Normalization Test: A New Diagnostic Test for Dry Eyes," *Cornea*, Vol. 25, No. 10, December 2006.

[f] U. de Sanctis, C. Loiacono, L. Richiardi, D. Turco, B. Mutani, and F. M. Grignolo, "Sensitivity and Specificity of Posterior Corneal Elevation Measured by Pentacam in Discriminating Keratoconus/Subclinical Keratoconus," *Ophthalmology*, Vol. 115, No. 9, September 2008.

[g] R. H. Silverman, R. Urs, A. RoyChoudhury, T. J. Archer, M. Gobbe, and D. Z. Reinstein, "Combined Tomography and Epithelial Thickness Mapping for Diagnosis of Keratoconus," *European Journal of Ophthalmology*, Vol. 27, No. 2, March 10, 2017.

[h] T. Kojima, N. Isogai, T. Nishida, T. Nakamura, and K. Ichikawa, "Screening of Keratoconus Using Autokeratometer and Keratometer Keratoconus Index," *Diagnostics*, Vol. 11, No. 11, November 15, 2021.

[i] A. Salman, T. Darwish, A. Ali, M. Ghabra, and R. Shaaban, "Sensitivity and Specificity of Sirius Indices in Diagnosis of Keratoconus and Suspect Keratoconus," *European Journal of Ophthalmology*, Vol. 32, No. 2, March 2022.

[j] P. M. Cumberland, A. Chianca, J. S. Rahi/UK Biobank Eye and Vision Consortium, "Accuracy and Utility of Self-Report of Refractive Error," *JAMA Ophthalmology*, Vol. 134, No. 7, July 2016.

[k] J. F. Leone, P. Mitchell, I. G. Morgan, A. Kifley, and K. A. Rose, "Use of Visual Acuity to Screen for Significant Refractive Errors in Adolescents: Is It Reliable?" *Archives of Ophthalmology*, Vol. 128, No. 7, July 2010.

[l] K. C. LaMattina, A. Vagge, and L. B. Nelson, "Can the Red Reflex Test Detect Unequal Refractive Error? *Journal of Pediatrics*, Vol. 214, November 2019.

[m] S. Marmamula, J. E. Keeffe, S. Narsaiah, R. C. Khanna, and G. N. Rao, "Population-Based Assessment of Sensitivity and Specificity of a Pinhole for Detection of Significant Refractive Errors in the Community," *Clinical and Experimental Optometry*, Vol. 97, No. 6, November 2014.

[n] A. R. Hathibelagal, P. Bhutia, M. Das, H. Babu, S. Jalali, B. Takkar, D. C. Paremeswarappa, and S. Ballae Ganeshrao, "Tablet-Based 'ON/OFF' Pathway Test Can Distinguish Between Rod- and Cone-Dominated Diseases," *Ophthalmic and Physiological Optics*, Vol. 43, No. 2, March 2023.

[o] A. C. Barnes, A. M. Hanif, and N. Jain, "Pentosan Polysulfate Maculopathy Versus Inherited Macular Dystrophies: Comparative Assessment with Multimodal Imaging," *Ophthalmology Retina*, Vol. 4, No. 12, December 2020.

[p] G. K. Frampton, N. Kalita, L. Payne, J. Colquitt, and E. Loveman, "Accuracy of Fundus Autofluorescence Imaging for the Diagnosis and Monitoring of Retinal Conditions: A Systematic Review," *Health Technology Assessment*, Vol. 20, No. 3, April 2016.

[q] N. H. Saliman, A. Belli, and R. J. Blanch, "Afferent Visual Manifestations of Traumatic Brain Injury," *Journal of Neurotrauma*, Vol. 38, No. 20, October 15, 2021.

[r] F. Topouzis, A. L. Coleman, F. Yu, L. Mavroudis, E. Anastasopoulos, A. Koskosas, T. Pappas, S. Dimitrakos, and M. R. Wilson, "Sensitivity and Specificity of the 76-Suprathreshold Visual Field Test to Detect Eyes with Visual Field Defect by Humphrey Threshold Testing in a Population-Based Setting: The Thessaloniki Eye Study," *American Journal of Ophthalmology*, Vol. 137, No. 3, March 2004.

[s] S. Bamdad, V. Beigi, and M. R. Sedaghat, "Sensitivity and Specificity of Swedish Interactive Threshold Algorithm and Standard Full Threshold Perimetry in Primary Open-Angle Glaucoma," *Medical Hypothesis, Discovery and Innovation in Ophthalmology*, Vol. 6, No. 4, Winter 2017.

To inform the model, we reviewed 24 articles to obtain the estimates of input parameters, sensitivity, and specificity. We then calculated the upper and lower bounds of the distribution of estimates we extracted from the literature, shown in Table 3.2. However, as illustrated in Table 2.7, some of these numbers, such as the lower bound of sensitivity for RE and the lower bounds of specificity for RE, dry eye, and glaucoma, have been modified based on the SME opinion. The sensitivity lower bound for RE increased to 0.7, and specificity lower bounds for dry eye, RE, and glaucoma increased to 0.7. Similarly, we modified the specificity upper bounds for all of the conditions, except for glaucoma, based on SME opinions. All these numbers changed to 0.98.

Abbreviations

AOA	American Optometric Association
CBA	cost-benefit analysis
CEA	cost-effectiveness analysis
DoD	Department of Defense
LHS	Latin hypercube sampling
NDRI	National Defense Research Institute
NMB	net monetary benefit
NSRD	National Security Research Division
OUSD	Office of the Under Secretary of Defense
OVD	ocular and visual dysfunction
P&R	Personnel and Readiness
PRCC	partial rank correlation coefficient
RE	refractive error
RF	risk factor
RMC	Regular Military Compensation
RYG	readiness years gained
SIPP	Survey of Income and Program Participation
SM	service member
SME	subject matter expert
TBI	traumatic brain injury
VDTBI	ocular and visual dysfunction secondary to traumatic brain injury
YOS	years of service

References

Alvarez, T. L., E. H. Kim, V. R. Vicci, S. K. Dhar, B. B. Biswal, and A. M. Barrett, "Concurrent Vision Dysfunctions in Convergence Insufficiency with Traumatic Brain Injury," *Optometry and Vision Science*, Vol. 89, No. 12, December 2012.

American Optometric Association, *Comprehensive Adult Eye and Vision Examination: Evidence-Based Clinical Practice Guidelines*, 2nd ed., 2022.

Amplify EyeCare, "How Much Does Keratoconus Treatment Cost?" undated. As of April 20, 2023: https://amplifyeye.care/article/how-much-does-keratoconus-treatment-cost/

AOA—*See* American Optometric Association.

Arnalich-Montiel, F., J. L. Hernández-Verdejo, N. Oblanca, F. J. Muñoz-Negrete, and M. P. De Miguel, "Comparison of Corneal Haze and Visual Outcome in Primary DSAEK Versus DSAEK Following Failed DMEK," *Graefe's Archive for Clinical and Experimental Ophthalmology*, Vol. 251, No. 11, November 2013.

Arnalich-Montiel, F., D. Mingo-Botín, and P. de Arriba-Palomero, "Preoperative Risk Assessment for Progression to Descemet Membrane Endothelial Keratoplasty Following Cataract Surgery in Fuchs Endothelial Corneal Dystrophy," *American Journal of Ophthalmology*, Vol. 208, December 2019.

Baker, N. D., H. S. Barnebey, M. R. Moster, M. C. Stiles, S. D. Vold, A. K. Khatana, B. E. Flowers, D. S. Grover, N. G. Strouthidis, J. F. Panarelli/INN005 Study Group, "Ab-Externo MicroShunt Versus Trabeculectomy in Primary Open-Angle Glaucoma: One-Year Results from a 2-Year Randomized, Multicenter Study," *Ophthalmology*, Vol. 128, No. 12, December 2021.

Bamdad, S., V. Beigi, and M. R. Sedaghat, "Sensitivity and Specificity of Swedish Interactive Threshold Algorithm and Standard Full Threshold Perimetry in Primary Open-Angle Glaucoma," *Medical Hypothesis, Discovery and Innovation in Ophthalmology*, Vol. 6, No. 4, Winter 2017.

Barnes, A. C., A. M. Hanif, and N. Jain, "Pentosan Polysulfate Maculopathy Versus Inherited Macular Dystrophies: Comparative Assessment with Multimodal Imaging," *Ophthalmology Retina*, Vol. 4, No. 12, December 2020.

Belviranli, S., and R. Oltulu, "Efficacy of Pulsed-Light Accelerated Crosslinking in the Treatment of Progressive Keratoconus: Two-Year Results," *European Journal of Ophthalmology*, Vol. 30, No. 6, November 2020.

Bourges, J.-L., "Corneal Dystrophies," *Journal français d'ophtalmologie*, Vol. 40, No. 6, June 2017.

Buckingham, R. S., L. L. Cornforth, K. J. Whitwell, and R. B. Lee, "Visual Acuity, Optical, and Eye Health Readiness in the Military," *Military Medicine*, Vol. 168, No. 3, March 2003.

Buckingham, R. S., D. McDuffie, K. Whitwell, and R. B. Lee, "Follow-Up Study on Vision Health Readiness in the Military," *Military Medicine*, Vol. 168, No. 10, October 2003.

Buckingham, R. S., K. J. Whitwell, and R. B. Lee, "Cost Analysis of Military Eye Injuries in Fiscal Years 1988–1998," *Military Medicine*, Vol. 170, No. 3, March 2005.

Chawla, H., and V. Vohra, "Retinal Dystrophies," StatPearls, last updated March 16, 2023. As of April 15, 2024:
https://www.ncbi.nlm.nih.gov/books/NBK564379/

Cumberland, P. M., A. Chianca, J. S. Rahi/UK Biobank Eye and Vision Consortium, "Accuracy and Utility of Self-Report of Refractive Error," *JAMA Ophthalmology*, Vol. 134, No. 7, July 2016.

CVS, "How Much Do Contacts Cost?" undated. As of April 20, 2023:
https://www.cvs.com/optical/article/how-much-do-contacts-cost

Dandona, R., L. Dandona, T. J. Naduvilath, M. Srinivas, C. A. McCarty, and G. N. Rao, "Refractive Errors in an Urban Population in Southern India: The Andhra Pradesh Eye Disease Study," *Investigative Ophthalmology and Visual Science*, Vol. 40, No. 12, November 1999.

De Sanctis, U., C. Loiacono, L. Richiardi, D. Turco, B. Mutani, and F. M. Grignolo, "Sensitivity and Specificity of Posterior Corneal Elevation Measured by Pentacam in Discriminating Keratoconus/Subclinical Keratoconus," *Ophthalmology*, Vol. 115, No. 9, September 2008.

Dhaliwal, D. K., V. Chirikov, J. Schmier, S. Rege, and S. Newton, "Cost Burden of Endothelial Keratoplasty in Fuchs Endothelial Dystrophy: Real-World Analysis of a Commercially Insured US Population (2014–2019)," *Clinical Ophthamology*, Vol. 16, April 6, 2022.

DoD—*See* U.S. Department of Defense.

DoD, OUSD(P&R)—*See* U.S. Department of Defense, Office of the Under Secretary of Defense for Personnel and Readiness.

El Afrit, M. A., D. Saadouli, G. Hachicha, K. Ben Mansour, N. El Afrit, and S. Yahyaoui, "The Outcome of Surgical Treatment in Advanced Glaucoma," *Archivos de la Sociedad Española de Oftalmología*, English ed., Vol. 96, No. 4, April 2021.

Eleiwa, T., A. Elsawy, M. Tolba, W. Feuer, S. Yoo, and M. A. Shousha, "Diagnostic Performance of 3-Dimensional Thickness of the Endothelium-Descemet Complex in Fuchs' Endothelial Cell Corneal Dystrophy," *Ophthalmology*, Vol. 127, No. 7, July 2020.

Fadlallah, A., A. Dirani, H. El Rami, G. Cherfane, and E. Jarade, "Safety and Visual Outcome of Visian Toric ICL Implantation After Corneal Collagen Cross-Linking in Keratoconus," *Journal of Refractive Surgery*, Vol. 29, No. 2, February 2013.

Frampton, G. K., N. Kalita, L. Payne, J. Colquitt, and E. Loveman, "Accuracy of Fundus Autofluorescence Imaging for the Diagnosis and Monitoring of Retinal Conditions: A Systematic Review," *Health Technology Assessment*, Vol. 20, No. 3, April 2016.

Frick, K. D., and E. L. Singman, "Cost of Military Eye Injury and Vision Impairment Related to Traumatic Brain Injury: 2001–2017," *Military Medicine*, Vol. 184, Nos. 5–6, 2019.

Gomes, J. A. P., P. F. Rodrigues, and L. L. Lamazales, "Keratoconus Epidemiology: A Review," *Saudi Journal of Ophthalmology*, Vol. 36, No. 1, July 11, 2022.

Gong, J., S. Cheung, A. Fasso-Opie, O. Galvin, L. S. Moniz, D. Earle, T. Durham, J. Menzo, N. Li, S. Duffy, J. Dolgin, et al., "The Impact of Inherited Retinal Diseases in the United States of America (US) and Canada from a Cost-of-Illness Perspective," *Clinical Ophthalmology*, Vol. 15, July 1, 2021.

Goodrich, G. L., H. M. Flyg, J. E. Kirby, C. Y. Chang, and G. L. Martinsen, "Mechanisms of TBI and Visual Consequences in Military and Veteran Populations," *Optometry and Vision Science*, Vol. 90, No. 2, February 2013.

Groth, L., B DeBroff, "How Much Does LASIK Eye Surgery Cost in 2024?" *Forbes Health*, 2024. As of May 16, 2024:
https://www.forbes.com/health/eye-health/how-much-does-lasik-cost/

Hathibelagal, A. R., P. Bhutia, M. Das, H. Babu, S. Jalali, B. Takkar, D. C. Paremeswarappa, and S. Ballae Ganeshrao, "Tablet-Based 'ON/OFF' Pathway Test Can Distinguish Between Rod- and Cone-Dominated Diseases," *Ophthalmic and Physiological Optics*, Vol. 43, No. 2, March 2023.

Health.mil, "Periodic Health Assessment," undated. As of July 26, 2023:
https://www.health.mil/Military-Health-Topics/Health-Readiness/Reserve-Health-Readiness-Program/Our-Services/PHA

Howell, A. H., "What's the Average Cost of a Cornea Transplant?" GoodRx, May 11, 2022. As of April 20, 2023:
https://www.goodrx.com/health-topic/eye/cornea-transplant-cost

Hwang, H. B., Y. H. Ku, E. C. Kim, H. S. Kim, M. S. Kim, and H. S. Hwang, "Easy and Effective Test to Evaluate Tear-Film Stability for Self-Diagnosis of Dry Eye Syndrome: Blinking Tolerance Time (BTT)," *BMC Ophthalmology*, Vol. 20, No. 1, November 2020.

Iman, R. L., J. C. Helton, and J. E. Campbell, "An Approach to Sensitivity Analysis of Computer Models: Part I—Introduction, Input Variable Selection and Preliminary Variable Assessment," *Journal of Quality Technology*, Vol. 13, No. 3, October 1981.

Ishak, K. J., N. Kreif, A. Benedict, and N. Muszbek, "Overview of Parametric Survival Analysis for Health-Economic Applications," *PharmacoEconomics*, Vol. 31, No. 8, August 2013.

Islam, S. S., E. J. Doyle, A. Velilla, C. J. Martin, and A. M. Ducatman, "Epidemiology of Compensable Work-Related Ocular Injuries and Illnesses: Incidence and Risk Factors," *Journal of Occupational and Environmental Medicine*, Vol. 42, No. 6, June 2000.

Johansson, J., C. Nygren de Boussard, G. Öqvist Seimyr, and T. Pansell, "The Effect of Spectacle Treatment in Patients with Mild Traumatic Brain Injury: A Pilot Study," *Clinical and Experimental Optometry*, Vol. 100, No. 3, May 2017.

Kojima, T., N. Isogai, T. Nishida, T. Nakamura, and K. Ichikawa, "Screening of Keratoconus Using Autokeratometer and Keratometer Keratoconus Index," *Diagnostics*, Vol. 11, No. 11, November 15, 2021.

Krull, Heather, Philip Armour, Kathryn A. Edwards, Kristin Van Abel, Linda Cottrell, and Gulrez Shah Azhar, "The Relationship Between Disability Evaluation and Accession Medical Standards," Santa Monica, Calif.: RAND Corporation, 2019. As of May 21, 2024:
https://www.rand.org/pubs/research_reports/RR2429.html

LaMattina, K. C., A. Vagge, and L. B. Nelson, "Can the Red Reflex Test Detect Unequal Refractive Error?" *Journal of Pediatrics*, Vol. 214, November 2019.

Latkany, R., B. G. Lock, and M. Speaker, "Tear Film Normalization Test: A New Diagnostic Test for Dry Eyes," *Cornea*, Vol. 25, No. 10, December 2006.

Leone, J. F., P. Mitchell, I. G. Morgan, A. Kifley, and K. A. Rose, "Use of Visual Acuity to Screen for Significant Refractive Errors in Adolescents: Is It Reliable?" *Archives of Ophthalmology*, Vol. 128, No. 7, July 2010.

Maguire, A. M., S. Russell, D. C. Chung, Z. F. Yu, A. Tillman, A. V. Drack, F. Simonelli, B. P. Leroy, K. Z. Reape, K. A. High, et al., "Durability of Voretigene Neparvovec for Biallelic RPE65-Mediated Inherited Retinal Disease: Phase 3 Results at 3 and 4 Years," *Ophthalmology*, Vol. 128, No. 10, October 2021.

Marmamula, S., J. E. Keeffe, S. Narsaiah, R. C. Khanna, and G. N. Rao, "Population-Based Assessment of Sensitivity and Specificity of a Pinhole for Detection of Significant Refractive Errors in the Community," *Clinical and Experimental Optometry*, Vol. 97, No. 6, November 2014.

Merezhinskaya, N., R. K. Mallia, D. Park, D. W. Bryden, K. Mathur, and F. M. Barker II, "Visual Deficits and Dysfunctions Associated with Traumatic Brain Injury: A Systematic Review and Meta-Analysis," *Optometry and Vision Science*, Vol. 96, No. 8, August 2019.

Merritt, Z. D., E. C. McNally, C. S. Allen, C. E. Bruff, G. A. Coleman, K. N. Harms, G. M. Mallie, C. W. Perdue, S. R. Putansu, T. L. Richardson, et al., *Military Personnel: Personnel and Cost Data Associated with Implementing DoD's Homosexual Conduct Policy*, Government Accountability Office, GAO-11-170, 2011.

Munir, S. Z., W. M. Munir, and J. Albrecht, "Estimated Prevalence of Keratoconus in the United States from a Large Vision Insurance Database," *Eye and Contact Lens: Science and Clinical Practice*, Vol. 47, No. 9, September 2021.

Musch, D. C., L. M. Niziol, J. D. Stein, R. M. Kamyar, and A. Sugar, "Prevalence of Corneal Dystrophies in the United States: Estimates from Claims Data," *Investigative Ophthalmology and Visual Science*, Vol. 52, No. 9, September 1, 2011.

National Eye Institute, "Glaucoma Tables," last updated February 7, 2020. As of April 17, 2024: https://www.nei.nih.gov/learn-about-eye-health/eye-health-data-and-statistics/glaucoma-data-and -statistics/glaucoma-tables

Nirwan, R. S., T. A. Albini, J. Sridhar, H. W. Flynn Jr., and A. E. Kuriyan, "Assessing 'Cell Therapy' Clinics Offering Treatments of Ocular Conditions Using Direct-to-Consumer Marketing Websites in the United States," *Ophthamology*, Vol. 126, No. 10, October 2019.

Oden, N. L., D. E. Lilienfeld, M. A. Lemp, J. D. Nelson, and F. Ederer, "Sensitivity and Specificity of a Screening Questionnaire for Dry Eye," *Advances in Experimental Medicine and Biology*, Vol. 438, 1998.

Paretts, Susan, "Glaucoma Surgery Cost and Financing," CareCredit, November 3, 2022.

Pinto-Bonilla, J. C., A. del Olmo-Jimeno, F. Llovet-Osuna, and E. Hernández-Galilea, "A Randomized Crossover Study Comparing Trehalose/Hyaluronate Eyedrops and Standard Treatment: Patient Satisfaction in the Treatment of Dry Eye Syndrome," *Therapeutics and Clinical Risk Management*, Vol. 11, April 13, 2015.

Rein, D. B., J. S. Wittenborn, P. Zhang, F. Sublett, P. A. Lamuda, E. A. Lundeen, and J. Saaddine, "The Economic Burden of Vision Loss and Blindness in the United States," *Ophthalmology*, Vol. 129, No. 4, April 2022.

Rein, D. B., P. Zhang, K. E. Wirth, P. P. Lee, T. J. Hoerger, N. McCall, R. Klein, J. M. Tielsch, S. Vijan, and J. Saaddine, "The Economic Burden of Major Adult Visual Disorders in the United States," *Archives of Ophthalmology*, Vol. 124, No. 12, December 2006.

Richards, S. J., "A Handbook of Parametric Survival Models for Actuarial Use," *Scandinavian Actuarial Journal*, Vol. 2012, No. 4, 2012.

Rotenstreich, Y., D. Harats, A. Shaish, E. Pras, and M. Belkin, "Treatment of a Retinal Dystrophy, Fundus albipunctatus, with Oral 9-cis-{beta}-Carotene. *British Journal of Ophthalmology*, Vol. 94, No. 5, May 2010.

Saliman, N. H., A. Belli, and R. J. Blanch, "Afferent Visual Manifestations of Traumatic Brain Injury," *Journal of Neurotrauma*, Vol. 38, No. 20, October 15, 2021.

Salman, A., T. Darwish, A. Ali, M. Ghabra, and R. Shaaban, "Sensitivity and Specificity of Sirius Indices in Diagnosis of Keratoconus and Suspect Keratoconus," *European Journal of Ophthalmology*, Vol. 32, No. 2, March 2022.

Scutti, S., "Gene Therapy for Rare Retinal Disorder to Cost $425,000 per Eye," CNN, January 2, 2018. As of April 20, 2023:
https://www.cnn.com/2018/01/03/health/luxturna-price-blindness-drug-bn/index.html

Shtein, R. M., J. F. Shen, A. N. Kuo, K. M. Hammersmith, J. Y. Li, and M. P. Weikert, "Autologous Serum-Based Eye Drops for Treatment of Ocular Surface Disease: A Report by the American Academy of Ophthalmology," *Ophthalmology*, Vol. 127, No. 1, January 2020.

Silverman, R. H., R. Urs, A. RoyChoudhury, T. J. Archer, M. Gobbe, and D. Z. Reinstein, "Combined Tomography and Epithelial Thickness Mapping for Diagnosis of Keratoconus," *European Journal of Ophthalmology*, Vol. 27, No. 2, March 10, 2017.

Sridhar, M. S., C. J. Rapuano, C. B. Cosar, E. J. Cohen, and P. R. Laibson, "Phototherapeutic Keratectomy Versus Diamond Burr Polishing of Bowman's Membrane in the Treatment of Recurrent Corneal Erosions Associated with Anterior Basement Membrane Dystrophy," *Ophthalmology*, Vol. 109, No. 4, April 2002.

Stinnett, A. A., and J. Mullahy, "Net Health Benefits: A New Framework for the Analysis of Uncertainty in Cost-Effectiveness Analysis," *Medical Decision Making*, Vol. 18, No. 2, Suppl., April 1998.

Topouzis, F., A. L. Coleman, F. Yu, L. Mavroudis, E. Anastasopoulos, A. Koskosas, T. Pappas, S. Dimitrakos, and M. R. Wilson, "Sensitivity and Specificity of the 76-Suprathreshold Visual Field Test to Detect Eyes with Visual Field Defect by Humphrey Threshold Testing in a Population-Based Setting: The Thessaloniki Eye Study," *American Journal of Ophthalmology*, Vol. 137, No. 3, March 2004.

Trieu, L. H., and J. B. Lavrich, "Current Concepts in Convergence Insufficiency," *Current Opinion in Ophthalmology*, Vol. 29, No. 5, September 2018.

U.S. Department of Defense, *Medical Standards for Military Service: Appointment, Enlistment, or Induction*, Department of Defense Instruction 6130.03, Vol. 1, November 16, 2022.

U.S. Department of Defense, Office of the Actuary, *Valuation of the Medicare-Eligible Retiree Health Care Fund*, January 2022. As of July 18, 2023:
https://actuary.defense.gov/Portals/15/MERHCF%20Val%20Report%202020.pdf?ver=nZyYW4h4H9N8i3rfLraz0w%3d%3d

U.S. Department of Defense, Office of the Under Secretary of Defense for Personnel and Readiness, Directorate of Compensation, *Selected Military Compensation Tables [Green Book]*, January 1, 2023, As of June 2, 2023: https://militarypay.defense.gov/Portals/3/GreenBook%202023.pdf

Vitale, S., L. Ellwein, M. F. Cotch, F. L. Ferris III, and R. Sperduto, "Prevalence of Refractive Error in the United States, 1999–2004," *Archives of Ophthalmology*, Vol. 126, No. 8, August 2008.

Walline, J. J., "Myopia Control: A Review," *Eye and Contact Lens*, Vol. 41, No. 1, January 2016.

Yim, C. K., A. Dave, A. Strawn, J. Chan, I. Zhou, and D. C. Zhu, "Visual Outcomes and Patient Satisfaction After Bilateral Refractive Lens Exchange with a Trifocal Intraocular Lens in Patients with Presbyopia," *Ophthalmology and Therapy*, Vol. 12, No. 3, June 2023.

Yu, J., C. V. Asche, and C. J. Fairchild, "The Economic Burden of Dry Eye Disease in the United States: A Decision Tree Analysis," *Cornea*, Vol. 30, No. 4, April 2011.